POLESAPART

A CHRISTIAN COUPLE GIVES BIPOLAR A VOICE

BY DR. ROBERT & JENNY BAKSS

Ark House Press
PO Box 1722, Port Orchard, WA 98366 USA
PO Box 1321, Mona Vale NSW 1660 Australia
PO Box 318 334, West Harbour, Auckland 0661 New Zealand
arkhousepress.com

All Scripture quotations are taken from the King James Version.
Special emphasis in verses is added.

First published in 2016 by Ark House Press
Distributed by Lighthouse Bookstore
A ministry of Lighthouse Baptist Church, Rockhampton
Lighthouse Bookstore, 480 Norman Road, Norman Gardens, QLD 4701,Australia
+61 7 4928 6633
bookstore@lighthousebaptist.com.au

The authors and publication team have put forth every effort to give proper credit to
quotes and thoughts that are not original with the authors. It is not our intent to claim
originality with any quote or thought that could not readily be tied to an original source.

For more resources on Poles Apart visit www.robertbakss.com

Cataloguing in Publication Data:
Title: Poles Apart
ISBN: 978-0-9953917-6-5 (pbk.)
Subjects: Mental Health, Healing, Christian Living
Other Authors/Contributors: Bakss, Robert

"Woman With No Mouth" was painted by artist Nina Neher from Rockhampton, Australia.
Cover design: Benjamin Bakss
Layout by initiateagency.com

To our precious children – Benjamin, Anna, Joshua, Timothy and Jonathan (JJ) – who have loved their mother unconditionally and supported her.

To our daughters-in-law and son-in-law - Alice, Kristy and Steve – who have been so understanding of our family dynamics and loved our children and been there for them during difficult times.

To our beautiful grandchildren – Mia, Caleb, Silas, Noah, Gracelyn, Annaliese, Marlia, Mikani and Jaylee – who have always brought great joy in our lives no matter what state we are in.

To our parents - Tom and Barbara and Lani - who have loved us with a tireless unconditional love and shown that love throughout our journey.

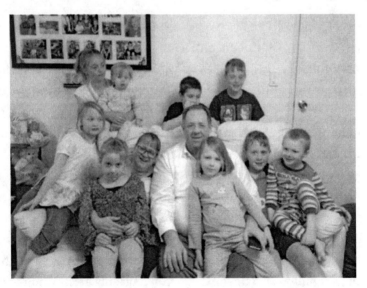

Robert and Jenny surrounded by their grandchildren.

ENDORSEMENTS

Incredibly inspiring and motivational – *Poles Apart* not only helps to remove the stigma of mental illness in our churches and society, it serves as an amazing witness and testimony for anyone with or without a mental illness. Thank you Robert and Jenny for opening the door of your life to the world by sharing your story and demonstrating your faith in God in a real, authentic and practical way. This book will definitely serve as an exceptional tool in my own practice and is a valuable resource within the mental health profession.

Barbara Wojtas, Adv.Dip.Couns., MACA
Counsellor and Family Therapist

Poles Apart by Dr Robert and Jenny Bakss provides an intimate glimpse into the reality of living with bipolar disorder; both from the perspective of the person with the condition and those sharing life with them. It perfectly captures the essence and dynamic of this multifaceted and often misunderstood illness, whilst dispelling myths and clarifying common misconceptions. The straightforward language ensures that even those without a medical background will be able to gain insight into the condition's complexity and the inherent dangers of failing to comply with a multi-disciplinary management strategy. As a natural health practitioner, I all too frequently meet people in search of a 'natural alternative', and emotions often run high when I attempt to explain the dangers of replacing a neurotransmitter modulating drug with herbal supplements. Only through increased awareness will misconceptions about acceptable treatment options be elucidated, and I believe 'Poles Apart' will play a fundamental role in this regard. I know this book will be a blessing to many and I wish Robert and Jenny all the best with their ongoing journey.

Dr Liza Pretorius DHM (UJ)
Natural Health Practitioner, Johannesburg, South Africa

With courage, empathy, and clarity, Robert and Jenny have eloquently shared their experience with bipolar disorder. While some have denied it and others have demonized it, Robert and Jenny have humbly brought mental illness into the light. They strike a marvellous balance detailing the profound struggles mental illness presents without excusing the many temptations mental illness brings. Although the book is not intended to be a medical resource, the reader will nonetheless find himself much better educated on the topic of bipolar affective disorder by the time he devours its pages. Perhaps most compelling of all is the steady theme of God's grace and goodness throughout each chapter. Truly the Lord has been faithful to strengthen, sustain, and now use as spokesmen this dear couple in the too often silent world of mental illness. Each of us knows someone who will benefit tremendously from this book. In some cases, it can literally be a life saver. It was my benefit to read it and my honour to recommend it now to you.

Pastor Kurt Skelly
Natrona Heights, Pennsylvania, USA

Thank you Dr. Robert and Jenny Bakss for your transparency in this powerful book, *Poles Apart*. In this book, Robert and Jenny Bakss describe the effects of bipolar disorder and use God's Word to help us better understand it. This book is very informative and will be helpful to those who have a desire to offer hope to anyone who suffers with bipolar disorder. Robert and Jenny have done an amazing job in telling their story and I can truly attest from their witness that Christ offers profound healing and hope for those wrestling with bipolar disorder.

Pastor Eric Capaci
Hot Springs, Arkansas, USA

TABLE OF CONTENTS

PART 3 – Therapies to Learn

AUTHORS NOTE BY ROBERT

This book was born from the unique personal experiences of Jenny and me. In telling our story, we recall events and raise issues from both of our perspectives. In order to avoid narrator confusion we have sought to identify who is writing at various points throughout the book. We utilised the following arrangement: 'I (Jenny)' to indicate where Jenny is the author, 'I (Robert)' to indicate where I am the author and at times when both of us are speaking, the narrative shifts to 'we'. There are times within the context of the book where the narrative uses the words 'we', 'you' and 'us' referring to every reader.

We have attempted to discuss issues relating to bipolar from both the perspective of the sufferer and from the one who loves and lives with the sufferer.

While many recollections of past events are clear, neither of us claims to have a photographic memory. We've reconstructed quotes and dialogue as accurately as possible to capture the essence of the moments as we recall them.

The book is not intended to be a reference text book on the subject of bipolar but rather our personal story living with this illness. It is for this reason we have used as few technical terms as possible and referred only to medical research where we felt it necessary to support our opinion and conclusions.

As Christians, we have relied on the Bible as our source for relevant scripture to help in providing advice and suggested actions. In some of the scripture verses quoted throughout the book, we have bolded certain words or phrases for emphasis.

The information in this book is intended to complement, not substitute for, the advice of your general practitioner, psychiatrist, psychologist or other mental health professionals who you should consult about your personal and unique needs. This book does not contain all-encompassing or comprehensive information regarding bipolar disorder and is not to be used or relied upon for any diagnostic or treatment purposes.

ACKNOWLEDGEMENTS

We are grateful to Margaret Gorle, Leanne Gray, Lana Gray, Lesley Henry, Barbara Wojtas and Lorraine McLeod who read through the manuscript at several stages, correcting our grammar, spotting the typos and offering suggestions – Thank you.

To Pastor Doug Fisher and his wife Patti who have given us counsel and support over the years – Thank you.

We thank the Lord for our friends in the ministry who have encouraged us, prayed for us and helped us during our journey. I (Robert) especially acknowledge the cards, text messages, emails, visits and gifts given to Jenny throughout her times of illness. Thank you to Eric and Carolann Capaci, Paul and Terrie Chappell, Steve and Lisa Chappell, Tim and Rebecca Cruse, James and Elisabet Felipe, David and Glorianne Gibbs Jr, Nathan and Cassie Lloyd, John and Gwen Nordman, Jeremy and Liz Pinero, Wayne and Suzanne Sehmish, Clarence and Evelyn Sexton, Kurt and Wanda Skelly, Josh and Heather Teis, Mark and Christine Tossell, Mansour and Sharon Youssef and Bill and Joseline Zaydan.

Thank you to our various church deacons and their wives who have served in that office throughout the years and supported and encouraged us along the way: Gary and Coral Ruff, Andrew and Barbara Wojtas, Ian and Leanne Gray and recently, Steve and Helena Bleakley.

Thank you my (Robert) associate pastors and their wives: John and Heather Buchholz and Mario and Alison Favari, who have supported and assisted me by stepping in to areas of ministry whenever I was unable to fulfil my obligations whilst caring for Jenny.

We acknowledge the help of our son Ben Bakss, Chris Gorle and Mina van der Colff who helped with the design, layout and website – Thank you.

To loyal, trusted and faithful friends who have been a pillar of strength and support in recent years: Jason Korda and Jeanne Harp - Thank you and may God bless you.

I (Jenny) acknowledge and thank my dear friends who personally understand bipolar and share our life experiences together: Ally Stegman and Terri Genocchio.

We appreciate the diligent and professional medical care received from Dr Sandy Prasad, Dr Lynne Steele, Dr John Flanagan, Dr Phillip Esdale, Dr Mary Russell and the patient, helpful and supportive assistance from all staff at the Hillcrest Archerview clinic.

Lastly, to the staff and church family at Lighthouse Baptist Church, we thank you for the constant love, care, prayers and support you all have shown to us both.

FRONT COVER PAINTING EXPLANATION

"Woman With No Mouth" was painted by artist Nina Neher from Rockhampton, Australia.

We asked Nina if she would paint an image for our book and gave her the brief and a snapshot of Jenny. The painting "Woman With No Mouth" was the creation of her artistic flare and personal understanding of the struggle with mental illness.

The woman is trying to express herself but has no mouth to form the words that reside deep within. She has been silenced by stigma, shame and insecurity. This is the story of many sufferers of mental illness.

The eyes cry out the soulish yearnings of those who desperately desire people to understand their plight while living with bipolar.

Thank you, Nina, for capturing the essence of the heart and emotion of our book.

Robert and Jenny Bakss

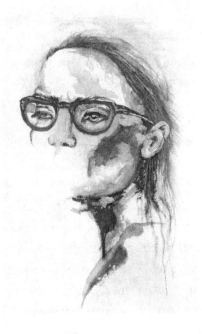 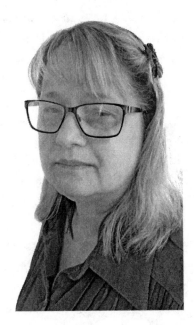

FOREWORD

BY DR SANDY PRASAD FRACGP, MBBS.

A s I open the door of my consultation room and exit into the waiting room beyond, I scan the sea of patients for a familiar face. I call Jenny's name and watch her rise, a kindly smile gracing her radiant face. It is not until we are both comfortably seated in my room and I ask her, "How are you going, Jenny?" that she gives a shy smile as she mumbles softly "Not so good, Sandy, not so good."

Just like Christian in John Bunyan's Pilgrim's Progress, I have seen this brave woman soldier on. I have seen her almost sink in the slough of despond only to be rescued by her loving family, friends and church members; I have seen her face and overcome the hill of difficulty. I have watched her battle Apollyon in the Valley of Humiliation, attacking not with her own strength but with the full armour of God. Most symbolically, I have seen her locked in doubting castle by the Giant Despair, whose booming voice tempted her, pressured her to take her life, to end it all and stop the suffering. But like Christian and Hopeful, though weak, weary and worn, she persevered. Like them, when she was brought to her knees and called out to God, she found that she had the key all along – the key to escaping the clutches of this fearsome giant. She discovered that Jesus Christ is the key, not just to freedom from her present troubles but to eternal life, so that she can be counted as one of those women who are worth far more than rubies, about whom through the grace of the Lord we may say with confidence: "*Strength and honour are her clothing; and she shall rejoice in time to come.*" (Proverbs 31:25)

Depression, bipolar, schizophrenia – these are serious medical conditions, just like diabetes. Just as the pancreas can have problems producing insulin, the brain can have chemical imbalances too. Mental conditions are not a curse or demonic possession, but a serious medical condition, which is as real as, and requires as much attention and action as, a problem with any other organ. Nevertheless, these people are not exempt from God's blessing, but rather experience the full glory of God in their lives when they decide to trust him, so that *"they that wait upon the LORD shall renew their strength; they shall mount up with wings as eagles; they shall run, and not be weary; and they shall walk, and not faint."(Isaiah 40:31)* Such is the destiny of beautiful people like Jenny.

PREFACE

Having bipolar disorder is like going to bed at night and waking up the next morning not knowing whether Tigger or Eeyore will be making your decisions for you.

It was during a stay in hospital at Archerview Mental Health Clinic where a good friend of mine, Ally, who also suffers from bipolar, first told me about Tigger and Eeyore. We both laughed and sighed knowing the absolute truth of the satirical pun.

I (Jenny) have been diagnosed with bipolar and have lived with it for twenty-three years as at the time of writing this book. The medical profession has labelled my condition as bipolar 1 disorder. This means I have extreme mood swings that at times create a euphoric, energetic person; at other times I don't have the energy to even get out of bed and simply curl up in the foetal position.

A few years ago it struck me, after hearing that up to forty-five percent of Australians will experience some sort of mental health condition in their lifetime, that maybe God has a purpose in this illness. Being a Christian woman struggling, managing, enduring and at times, as weird as it may sound, rejoicing in this illness, I and my husband Robert believed it might be a help to others to know of our journey through life with this third companion called, 'bipolar'.

It is our prayer and hope that the lessons God and others have taught us and what we have learned through the highs and lows will bring a measure of hope, blessing and encouragement to sufferers of bipolar and other mental illnesses, along with those who live with, care for, support and know them.

As a spouse of a person living with bipolar, I (Robert) have and still am learning to minister with and exercise compassion and mercy. In essence, those who are not afflicted with a mental illness must help bear the burden of those who have an unanswered prayer – the prayer to be rid of the illness. In Jenny's case she has prayed and prayed for God to remove the infirmity - her 'thorn in the flesh'. The answer has been "no." My role as her husband is to help her and show compassion for her plight of living with an unanswered prayer. Jenny has come to understand the words of the apostle Paul in a greater way when he said:

> "And lest I should be exalted above measure through the abundance of the revelations, there was given to me a **thorn in the flesh**, the messenger of Satan to buffet me, lest I should be exalted above measure. For this thing I besought the Lord thrice, that it might depart from me. And he said unto me, **My grace is sufficient for thee**: for my strength is made **perfect in weakness**. Most gladly therefore will I rather glory in my infirmities, that the **power of Christ may rest upon me**. Therefore I take pleasure in infirmities, in reproaches, in necessities, in persecutions, in distresses for Christ's sake: for when I am weak, then am I strong." (2 Corinthians 12:7-10)

In my biased opinion, Jenny is a stronger woman because of her weakness and has the power of Christ resting upon her.

We desire these humble words on a page to aid in breaking the silence and stigma that surrounds mental illness within our society and especially within the Christian community.

Join us on our journey. Let's begin.

PART 1

TRIALS OF LIFE

CHAPTER 1

WHAT IS WRONG WITH ME?

DILEMMA

Throughout life there are times and circumstances when we want to believe that heaven can heal the sorrow and pain that people go through. However, the lingering health issue, the increasing marital struggles and worry over children or money end up keeping their souls tied in knots. Sometimes it feels like there are more questions than answers.

"Why, God? Why this? Why me? Why now?"

One thing weaves us all together into the same tapestry. It is the common thread of humanity and it comes in all shapes and sizes and various times and seasons. It is what we call suffering. We know suffering is inevitable but in the midst of it we long to see some rhyme or reason, some purposeful pattern, a design in the making.

When we look at a work of tapestry, it is a combination of woven pieces of coloured thread that are intricately placed according to the designer to form a beautiful piece of artwork. However, a glance at the back of the tapestry shows a far different picture. It often looks like nothing more than gnarled threads and missed stitches. From our earthly perspective, all we see is the back of the canvas of our life that God is intricately weaving together. As we look into the Word of God we will gain a glimpse of the heavenward side of that tapestry. This has been our story as a couple grappling with a Christian woman's journey with bipolar.

One hot summer's afternoon in December 1993 I (Jenny) had no energy and felt like I wanted to yell at the children for no particular reason. These feelings were just not me. My husband, Robert, was working at the time and when he got home from work he suggested I lie down and get some sleep. He said, "You'll feel better in the morning." Unfortunately, I never did.

We had no idea what was happening.

We had moved to Rockhampton, Queensland, in January of that year with our three children, Benjamin (7 years old), Anna (5 years old) and Joshua (3 years old). Robert had accepted the offer to become the Youth Pastor at Norman Park Baptist Church and also secured a job working in local government undertaking legal and administration functions.

We were beginning our ministry life together and were so excited. Every Friday night we would leave our youngest Joshua, with a dear elderly couple, Mr & Mrs Janes, while the rest of us would head to church for Friday night Kids' Club and Youth Group. Robert would drive the bus and pick up the youth and we would work with fifty or so young people. We enjoyed this immensely and felt God had given us a great ministry to impact these lives. The weekends were busy with home duties, Sunday school, church services and the occasional hospitality.

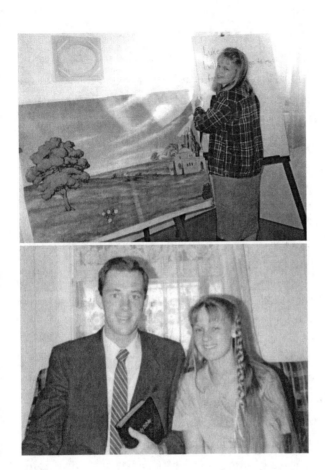

Top: Jenny teaching Sunday School

Below: Robert and Jenny serving the Lord

As a church, we were planning and getting ready to open a Christian School in 1994 and in the meantime we decided to home school Ben and Anna.

Our lives were busy, full and happy. Then entered the unwanted visitor in late 1993.

We had already had the stress-filled incident in December and things were not improving. I (Robert) came home from work to find Jenny completely frazzled and frustrated. I had never seen her look at me like this before. Her eyes were full of what seemed a mixture of fear, anger and confusion. Jenny looked at me and then ran and hurled herself at the dining room wall in her frustration, leaving her bruised and stunned. We sat there on the dining room floor holding each other and crying amidst the broken pieces of fibro wall sheeting. Bipolar mental illness became a resident in our home.

At this stage we had no idea what was happening. We knew nothing about mental illness and the subject of bipolar disorder.

What we were about to discover in the years to come was that Jenny was living a life poles apart!

The expression 'poles apart' often refers to people being very different or far from coming to an agreement with each other. It can also allude to the distance between the north and south poles. In fact, there is an unusual sea creature known as the sea butterfly that is considered to be bipolar, living in both the Arctic and Antarctic oceans. For the purposes of this book, 'poles apart' is a reference to the extreme, opposite moods experienced by a person living with bipolar disorder.

But what do you do when you have two poles inside of you? You are literally poles apart and yet one person in one place. That is the struggle of a person living with bipolar.

After the first major bipolar episode (though at the time we didn't know it was bipolar) Jenny became very depressed and subsequently suffered the sad and often tragic results of depression. Her loss of appetite caused her to lose 30% of her body weight over a period of six months. From a physically healthy 60 kilogram woman, Jenny became a weak and body-toneless 40 kilo frame. Whilst some would relish the idea of losing this much weight, this unwanted drop in weight affected her lifestyle and left her with very little strength. It wasn't just the body fat that diminished; it was loss of muscle vitality from the constant hours of sleep both day and night with little to no exercise.

Desires of life fled away like a boat sailing away into the distance over the horizon. I (Jenny) never thought I would be stable and 'normal' (whatever that is) again. To live with a constant brain fog is the best way to explain how my thoughts and mind felt.

Suicidal thoughts plagued me in the night time and lonely times of the day when Robert was at work. I would sit and ponder all the reasons my family would be better off without me and how I would no longer have the constant wrestling in my mind both day and night. Silence was literally deafening and yet noise was irritating.

Then, just like someone turning on a switch my mood would swing from very low to very high. These times I called my 'highs' or my 'good times'; and they would often be accompanied by some bizarre and at times expensive behaviours. During these episodes of 'highs', insomnia kicked in and I could literally go full steam for days without sleep.

It would be a few weeks later when some late night TV shopping channel parcels arrived that I (Robert) realised what Jenny had done during one of her sleepless 'high' nights - shopping sprees from the privacy of our own home!

During the 'highs', I (Jenny) would think irrational thoughts and begin working on grandiose plans for home improvements, gardening, sewing projects, ministry ideas and organising family gatherings and impromptu parties all in the space of 48 to 72 hours with no sleep. The dining room table became my designer's desk with materials and objects strewn all over the place, relegating family meals to the lounge room. I would have thoughts and ideas just racing through my head so fast that I would wonder if I could even catch up to myself.

We both soon learned that the highs, which were exhausting for everyone, were often a reprieve from the lows. We knew if there is an up, there usually is a down just around the corner. We were right! We would call these times 'the crash'.

It was difficult for family and friends to understand the dramatic swings. It was not uncommon for people to see Jenny in one of her highs or to receive a phone call from her during those times, then comment to me (Robert), "It's great to see Jenny doing so well." Little did they know that that morning Jenny had come down off the high. She had gone from insomnia to hypersomnia, or oversleeping and was in another 'crash' withdrawing from people and events. There is often a confused look on the faces of those who hear of the sudden change in behaviour and find it difficult to reconcile the 'two Jennys'.

When these lows hit me (Jenny), I feel lethargic. I just want to be left alone and depression clouds my mind. I've slipped into what I call the 'pit'.

It was in these moments I would ask myself and God, "What is happening to me?" I would wonder, "Am I going crazy?" I became swallowed up in my own negative thoughts and feelings and would say to Robert, "I just can't think".

I would have outbursts of anger and it was in these times when my children and my husband would get the brunt of all my negative thoughts and perceptions. Sadly, in my sadness and frustration I have said hurtful things to my family and especially to Robert, even accusing him of being a bad husband, father and pastor, which is far from the truth. But the 'pit' becomes my reality and blocks my view of the truth. Afterwards, when the anger subsides I feel so guilty about what I have said and how I have hurt people and I sink even deeper into the 'pit'. It's like I really am my own worst enemy.

More feelings of guilt and unworthiness would plague me, as a wife and mother, when I would go through periods of depression where I was literally numb with no feelings for my husband and children. The cuddles from the children and the tears would not move me or affect me. It was like something had died within me. I had gone from having a vibrant family life to all of a sudden being totally empty within. It was like a switch turned me off and I no longer reacted to anything. I'm thankful that Robert was understanding and patient with me in these times.

I would stay this way for sometimes up to a month or more and just couldn't bring myself out of the 'pit'. I would try to push myself and only end up further exhausted and shaking within and without. In the early years of my sickness, I would get tired of being trapped and this is when I had thoughts of self harm and suicide to escape the pain. I'm thankful I never attempted to carry out any of my thoughts of ending my life. I suppose I had come to realise I didn't really want to die: I just wanted to be 'normal' again.

I pleaded with God in prayer to take away this insanity and wept buckets of tears crying myself to sleep and sometimes lying awake on my drenched pillow.

Surely there must be a reason why I am like I am. I was so confused.

As a Christian, I knew I needed to seek solace from my Lord and Saviour, Jesus Christ and allow the Holy Spirit and His Word to become my comfort. Yet the 'pit' seemed so deep and dark that I felt like a trapped person stumbling for a light to show me the way back to God. Any time I read and pondered on the words of the Bible it seemed I always saw the negative and kept myself in the 'pit'.

Little did I realise then that the very Bible I struggled to pick up and read, and the very God who loved me unconditionally, would become my greatest source of hope in the darkest moments of life. The Lord certainly proved to me that He was there all the time and was true to His word: *"...for he hath said, I will never leave thee, nor forsake thee" (Hebrews 13:5).*

The words of the psalmist David would eventually become my mantra when, through my illness I came to know the Lord like I had never known Him before. In Psalm 139, David describes how God knows us in every detail and this became a truth that helped me in my trust of God no matter what was happening in my brain.

> *"O LORD, thou hast searched me, and known me. Thou knowest my downsitting and mine uprising, thou understandest my thought afar off. Thou compassest my path and my lying down, and art acquainted with all my ways. For there is not a word in my tongue, but, lo, O LORD, thou knowest it altogether. Thou hast beset me behind and before, and laid thine hand upon me. Such knowledge is too wonderful for me; it is high, I cannot attain unto it." (Psalm 139:1-6)*

The next part of the psalm reminded me that my Lord is always there and knows my name and every move I make. Even when I felt I just wanted to escape or hide, in a vain hope that everything would be stable again, He was still there! I didn't need to go anywhere; the destination and situation was not my problem. I simply had bipolar and God knew all about it, even before I was born.

> "Whither shall I go from thy spirit? or whither shall I flee from thy presence? If I ascend up into heaven, thou art there: if I make my bed in hell, behold, thou art there. If I take the wings of the morning, and dwell in the uttermost parts of the sea; Even there shall thy hand lead me, and thy right hand shall hold me. If I say, Surely the darkness shall cover me; even the night shall be light about me. Yea, the darkness hideth not from thee; but the night shineth as the day: the darkness and the light are both alike to thee. For thou hast possessed my reins: thou hast covered me in my mother's womb. I will praise thee; for I am fearfully and wonderfully made: marvellous are thy works; and that my soul knoweth right well. My substance was not hid from thee, when I was made in secret, and curiously wrought in the lowest parts of the earth. Thine eyes did see my substance, yet being unperfect; and in thy book all my members were written, which in continuance were fashioned, when as yet there was none of them." (Psalm 139:7-16)

I began to understand that God knew everything about me and what I needed to help me in life. This realisation gave me hope to trust in God whom I can talk to anytime and anywhere.

> "How precious also are thy thoughts unto me, O God! how great is the sum of them! If I should count them, they are more in number than the sand: when I awake, I am still with thee." (Psalm 139:17-18)

I have learned that even though I fight battles in my mind, it does not mean I have to lose the battle. My God is still with me and thinks upon me. I believe that He created my mind when He created my life. He didn't make a mistake.

This was to be part of my journey as a Christian woman living with what I would soon discover was bipolar disorder.

CHAPTER 2

MY ILLNESS HAS A NAME

DIAGNOSIS

"I don't really know what to do for your wife. Just take her to the Psychiatric Ward and leave her there. They might be able to figure it out". These were the words the first doctor told my husband when we were desperately seeking some answers.

Robert wasn't going to take me to the Psychiatric Ward and just leave me there. So we prayed, and begged God to lead us to someone who might be able to give us a diagnosis.

If you have ever had a mysterious illness or condition, you know there are often well-meaning family and friends who have read or seen something and have the diagnosis already worked out. In the early days of my illness, as sincere as they might be, everyone had opinions as to what was wrong with me and how I needed to fix it.

Trusted friends, who we knew loved us and wanted nothing more than to help find an answer, went in a quest to discover what was wrong with me. With the World Wide Web in its infancy the online solutions to medical issues were scarce and at times dubious. Nevertheless, they were available and amateur research became that much easier for those who were able to access the internet.

This led to several ideas as to why I was behaving so erratically and experiencing the highs and lows. We knew there was something going wrong in my thinking and at first some of the spiritual mentors and pastors in our life counselled me purely in the topics of fear, trust, prayer and faith in God. Whilst the verses of scripture and counsel were useful in helping me process some of my random thoughts, the mind games continued.

Some thought the real problem was having three young children and attempting to home school the two eldest and if I just put them in school all my problems would end. Others suggested the mental problems I had might be cured with a treatment for Candida, even though that wasn't really an issue. Still, others opted for more exercise and a selective brain food diet with a vitamin and supplement program. There were also the warnings to be on guard against the doctors who are 'in bed' with the prescription companies and to not be lulled into false medical advice. Many just simply said, "Get over it; snap out of it!". I even had a pastor slap me across the face and tell me, "Get over it and stop being silly."

Videos and later DVDs, together with books and magazine articles, soon came in the mail along with deliveries accompanied by a 'get well' card or a thoughtful caring note.

I must admit, it was tiring and mentally exhausting trying not to disappoint someone who really believed their solution would work.

After a while I felt somewhat like Job in the Bible when his friends were telling him what they thought was his problem and how he needed to correct it. He said to his three friends who came to console him in his loss, *"I have heard many such things: miserable comforters are ye all." (Job 16:2)*

My cycles of depression and hypermania were becoming more frequent and the hope of finding a balanced and 'normal life' was seemingly fading with time.

During the school holidays it became a regular occurrence for me and the children to stay with their grandparents on the Sunshine Coast (about an eight hour car trip from where we lived) while Robert had to continue to work in Rockhampton. Then when school holidays ended I would stay longer with my parents or with Robert's mother who would care for me, whilst Robert would get the kids settled back into the school routine. By this time, we had enrolled the children into our church Christian school which had opened within a couple of years of arriving in Rockhampton.

It was during one of these extended stays away that a break through came. I had been referred to a mental health doctor who was the first to suggest that I may have bipolar disorder and recommended a course of treatment. At last someone had given my journey a name! The doctor explained to us for the first time the impact of serotonin levels on the brain and how deficiency may be a cause of bipolar. Serotonin is a chemical your body produces that's needed for your nerve cells and brain to function.

It's helpful to have a name for what it is. There's a strange comfort you receive in naming an issue. It means you're not alone and other people are with you in this, even though your symptoms may not look like another person's.

We both began to read widely on the subject to understand it. We searched libraries and doctors' offices and yes, Google!

We learned that bipolar affective disorder, or more commonly known as bipolar disorder, (formerly known as manic depressive disorder) is a mental illness classified as a mood disorder. There are several forms of the disorder, some being more severe, while others emphasise either the mania or the depression side of the disorder. In general, the disorder is characterised by extreme highs and lows in mood which affect emotions, thoughts and behaviours. The manic episodes are what make this mood disorder different from other forms of depression. Mania can include any of the following symptoms: a feeling of inflated self-importance, grandiose thinking, hyper speech, racing thoughts, increased energy levels, risky behaviours and wildly unrealistic judgment. The manic-depressive is easily agitated or angered when these fantastic views inevitably meet reality. Thus, a manic episode is typically followed by an explosion of anger and a plunge into depression and despair.

I now discovered I have a possible chemical imbalance in my brain that makes it hard for my body to balance out my hormones. This is what causes such drastic changes in mood from the extreme highs to the deep lows and it is why I was diagnosed with a 'mood disorder.' To most of my friends and family, the announcement that I have bipolar disorder was greeted by confused stares and some tears. Nobody knew much about the illness and scepticism was in the air.

The diagnosis of bipolar disorder is a symptomatic diagnosis rather than a scientific one. No blood test, brain scan or any other medical test can confirm a person has bipolar. It is simply the result of examining the symptoms (evidence of an illness) and then making a diagnosis.

One problem that can occur with people like me, is they can be misdiagnosed as simply having depression. This is a problem in the treatment and management of the illness since anti-depressants alone don't treat the mood cycling and instability and not the mania episodes. An article in the Medical Journal of Australia stated,

"Delayed and incorrect diagnoses are common in bipolar disorder, and unipolar depression is a frequent misdiagnosis."[1]

With me, bipolar disorder was more than just a fleeting good or bad mood; the cycles of bipolar disorder last for days, weeks, or even months. The diagnosis was correct and I am now living with a mental illness called bipolar disorder.

Mental Health Australia defines a mental illness as follows:

> *Mental illness is a general term for a group of illnesses that affect the mind or brain. These illnesses, which include bipolar disorder, depression, schizophrenia, anxiety and personality disorders, affect the way a person thinks, feels and acts. The exact cause of mental illness is unknown. What is known is that mental illness is NOT a character fault, weakness or something inherently 'wrong' with a person. It is an illness like any other.*[2]

Information about bipolar wasn't as readily available then as it is today. However, armed with this information I was able to go back to my family doctor who continued me on a course of medication (Efexor) aimed to increase the serotonin levels and balance my hormones.

Medicine that targets brain chemistry is not an exact science and we have come to realise what works for one patient may not work for another. However, it started to work for me. Within a couple of weeks we began to see some dramatic improvements and I returned

---

1 'Diagnosis and monitoring of bipolar disorder in general practice', by Philip B Mitchell, Colleen K Loo and Bronwyn M Gould. 2010, Medical Journal of Australia. https://www.mja.com.au/journal/2010/193/4

2 https://mhaustralia.org/resources/frequently-asked-questions/what-mental-illness

to what seemed normalcy, which I hadn't been accustomed to for what seemed like years.

Doctors warned us of plenty: that medications can lose their effectiveness; that in time the illness may reoccur again and again; that this was a lifelong illness that needed to be managed for life; and that I would be on medication to balance my moods for the rest of my life.

That's okay with me because I know Who is really keeping me sane. The Lord is my balance.

As with other health conditions, mental illnesses are often physical as well as emotional and psychological. They may be caused by reactions to environmental stresses, genetic factors, biochemical imbalances or a combination of these. With the proper care and treatment, many people learn to manage and live with their illness and continue functioning in their daily lives. Mental illness is real and highly treatable.

CHAPTER 3

WHAT IS THIS THING CALLED BIPOLAR?

DEFINITIONS

Christmas time for most families is filled with a focus on the birth of Jesus, seasonal greetings and decorations, exchanging of gifts, and of course Christmas food and festivities. Over the years in our home, I (Jenny) have at times added some unique variations to our Christmas celebrations. On one occasion, after experiencing extremely high levels of energy, I slept less than two to four hours a night for the week leading up to Christmas Day. Very early on Christmas morning, while it was still dark, I woke everybody up, much to my teenagers' displeasure. I was full of excitement with the idea of a family photo and made them all put on the red T-shirts I had purchased the day before. My enthusiasm didn't seem too contagious at three o'clock in the morning!

Another time, my daughter-in-law Alice tells me of the time she came across my three eldest children (Benjamin, Anna and Joshua), who were tired and cranky as they began their day. The reason for their unfriendly disposition was because, following another sleepless high-energy night, I had woken them up very early to come outside and pick mangoes from our mango tree, even though they were still a little green. It was their grandmother's birthday and I thought it would be a great idea to have her grandchildren pick her some mangoes to go along with the birthday cake I had baked in the early morning hours. Admittedly, five o'clock in the morning on a school day was a bit much. But, I was on a high and loving it - the next morning I still didn't even feel tired.

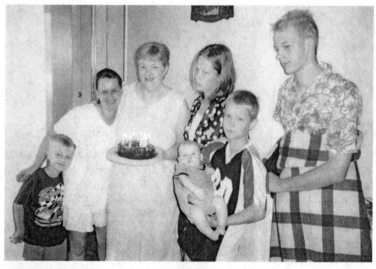

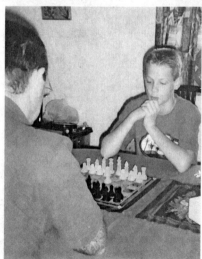

Above: The looks on the faces say it all!

Left: Red shirt day!

One Christmas was the complete opposite to what I described before. This time after months of pre-planning to host and organise the entire family Christmas lunch with around twenty-five guests invited, I slipped rapidly into a deep low of depression with added severe anxiety attacks and shakes. My bedroom became my refuge for several days, including Christmas Day and I had no desire to talk with anyone. Robert, our daughter Anna and daughters-in-law, Alice and Kristy, stepped in to rescue the day. Little did I know, Robert already had a back-up plan ready for when I would crash.

I was suffering from bipolar disorder, which has been described as one of the most perplexing and severe psychiatric mood disorders or adjustment conditions. The illness is one that, as in my case, can cause frustration, confusion, incredible suffering and uncertainty for the individual, friends and the family.

My cycles became more intense and frequent. After a prolonged period of an extreme low, where I had become dysfunctional, I was finally hospitalised to undergo electric shock treatment. I will talk more about that dark time further on in the book.

As I have already mentioned, bipolar disorder was formerly known as manic-depressive illness or manic depression and gets its name from the unpredictable emotional rollercoaster mood swings ranging from the pole of extreme highs (mania) to the pole of deep lows (depression). From my experience and research, people with bipolar disorder often spend more time in the depressive phase of illness than the manic phase. Between the fluctuating polar emotions called 'episodes' are the periods of balanced moods.

For those who have never experienced a mania episode, let me try to describe the euphoria you feel in the moment. Imagine a time in your life when you had an emotional high after a very pleasant, positive event. Maybe it was when you received an award and public recognition or a time when you had the proverbial stomach butterflies when falling in love. Perhaps the feeling was the exhilaration of reaching the top of a mountain you've climbed. Then multiply the intensity of that feeling three or four times, speed it up to 'fast forward,' triple your energy level and imagine feeling that way around the clock for days, even weeks until you collapse from

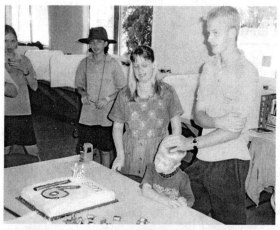

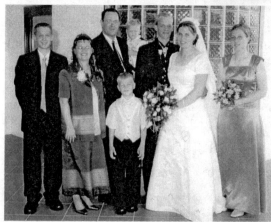

Above: Ben's 16th Birthday cake – four months late!

Below: Wedding day of Ben and Alice

exhaustion. This is a little of what a high or hypermania episode feels like. It begins with so much fun for me but ends with a deep dive into depression.

You might ask, "What's the problem with having so much energy and being on a high?" There are several dangers and unfortunate results that come from being at this end of the pole. Firstly, you are probably going to do a lot of exaggerated and unwise things during your manic state. Whilst they may seem humorous in hindsight, they can have disastrous effects at the time and afterwards.

On Anna's thirteenth birthday in May, I was unwell and unable to celebrate with her. So, during a high moment in the month of October, I decided to bring a birthday cake to her school and interrupt the class in session and ask the class to sing her Happy Birthday. This ill-timed expression of love created a slightly embarrassing moment for my daughter who later had to try to awkwardly explain my random bizarre acts to her classmates. The next year it was the same song second stanza but this time it was a cake for Ben's sixteenth birthday - four months late!

Weddings are wonderful events and as is the practice in Australia, the ceremony is followed by the wedding reception dinner with all the guests. As great as weddings are, they can also be very expensive and at times the guest list for the reception is often cut to fit within the budget constraints. Unless of course you are on a bipolar high! The first of our children to marry was our eldest son, Benjamin. I was definitely on a high leading up to this event which was evident in the days prior to the wedding when I was inviting random acquaintances to attend the wedding and even the reception. Robert had to follow up after my spree of invitations and clarify the late invitation was only to the ceremony and politely retract the invite to the reception.

Many people think a manic person is simply a very happy, high-energy, elated person and this is part of bipolar disorder that is often difficult to diagnose at first. Bipolar mania is more than normal mood fluctuations. When you are experiencing a high, you can become excessively elated, irritable, moody and energetic all at the same time. Your racing thoughts may lead you to begin a conversation and then jump abruptly to unrelated topics without any warning or transition.

Robert and I have known of some people in their high moments that are very easy to distract and seemingly act on every impulse. It is common to have an exaggerated sense of your own importance and be slightly over-confident about your abilities. Whilst in a state of mania, I can also become extremely outgoing and sociable. Close friends and family have told me I have even become the life of the party at times.

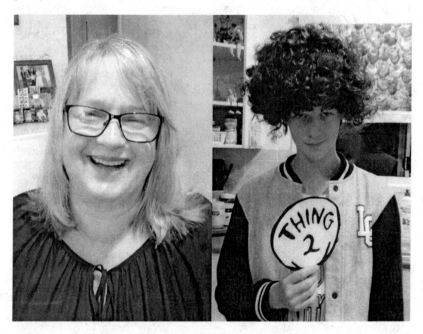

Happy day for Jenny but not so happy times for JJ with the dress up!

I (Robert) recall a time when we were about 12 years into the bipolar journey and Jenny and I were attending a Pastors and wives' marriage retreat. During a segment of the retreat we broke up for a time of separate instruction for men and women. I was assigned the task of teaching a session to the pastors whilst another lady was supposed to be teaching a session to the wives. However, earlier that day during a lunch break, Jenny and I headed out to do a little shopping. I knew something was brewing as I observed her mood becoming very elated. For example, we passed by a lingerie shop and Jenny impulsively decided to go in and buy several items whilst I was requested to embarrassingly stand by the dressing room and help make the choices. This was slightly out of character for Jenny and I wondered what would happen next. We headed back to the retreat and went into the split sessions. At the end of the sessions the couples all came back together for some afternoon tea. It was at this moment I soon realised what had happened, as some comments were made to me by some of the other wives that they found Jenny's contribution to the session 'interesting'. Jenny had a mania moment and decided to hand out a piece of paper to all the ladies present and kind of 'took over' the session asking a series of questions of the ladies who were instructed by her to write their answers down. From this event though, some of the ladies became aware that something wasn't right and instead of stigmatising Jenny, they became and have remained faithful friends who pray and express their care for her continual well-being.

The bad part about a high for a person suffering from bipolar is they end. When it does, you come crashing into deep depression. Sadly the statistics claim that 10 to 15 percent of people with bipolar disorder end up committing suicide especially after they have come down from a manic episode. Common thoughts like, "There's no hope" and "My mood swings just get worse and worse and I'll never have a normal life" are what many experience.

To somewhat understand the opposite pole of depression and an extreme low, just reverse the imagination to a sad moment or a time of discouragement and magnify the feeling ten times. What makes it even more intensely unbearable is that, unlike a normal period of sadness or discouragement, bipolar depression just hits you for no apparent reason. The search for a reason is often what sets the spiral going deeper and faster. You are frustrated and others keep asking you, "What set you off this time?" to which everything inside of you screams, "I don't know! I wish there was something, then I could deal with it!"

On one occasion when I (Jenny) was in a low, I was unable to tolerate any noise and became very agitated and extremely irritable. The sound of the television was annoying me and I had asked the children to not watch it. While the children were at school I had devised a plan to stop the television from ever working again. In a moment of frustration and poor judgement, I took a pair of scissors and cut the power cord in half to solve my noise dilemma. On arrival home from school our eldest son, Ben, discovered what I had done and decided to rectify the matter and ensure his bipolar mother wouldn't be able to destroy the television again. He found a piece of PVC pipe and re-ran the power cord inside it to protect it from my lethal scissors. After this event, I was affectionately nicknamed "Jenny Scissorhands" by some of my children and their friends.

Sometimes Christians in a manic phase may stop their regular responsibilities and intensely read the Bible or talk to one person after another about God for hours and hours. However, often for me, in the early years of my bipolar, I turned to the Bible for solace in my lows but only saw the negative in passages of scripture that seemed to condemn my heart even more. Christians in a depressed state typically feel incredibly guilty and self-condemning and may be convinced that God wouldn't or couldn't love them in the state they are in. It was during one of my very down moments, Pastor Doug Fisher from San Diego, a godly pastor and our personal friend, was able to counsel with me. His insight into the scripture coupled with his own personal testimony, from wrestling with depressive thoughts on a few occasions in life, became a source of light in the darkness. One verse of scripture he pointed me to was written by the apostle John to remind me God is greater than any self-condemnation. *"For if our heart condemn us, God is greater than our heart, and knoweth all things."* (1 John 3:20)

According to the American Psychiatric Association, the common symptoms of bipolar disorder[3] include emotional, cognitive, behavioural and physical changes such as:

Highs (Mania)

- Experiencing an elevated, euphoric, expansive or irritable mood
- Feeling excessively good about self (inflated self esteem)
- Exaggerated ideas about how important one is (grandiosity)
- Having many ideas or thoughts at the one time (flight of ideas)
- Speedy or racing thoughts
- Easily distracted or impulsive

---

3 Diagnostic and Statistical Manual of Mental Disorders, Fifth Edition (DSM-5) is the standard classification of mental disorders used by mental health professionals in the United States. It is intended to be used in all clinical settings by clinicians of different theoretical orientations. Washington, D.C 2013.

- Acting overly joyful or silly

- Having a short fuse or temper

- Expressing extreme agitation

- Thinking or talking rapidly

- Unusually talkative or feeling compelled to keep talking

- Sleeping very few hours without the side effect of fatigue

- Having sexual thoughts, discussions and behaviours more than usual

- Exhibiting unpredictable behaviour and impaired judgment

- Involvement in pleasurable or risky activities that have the potential for serious negative consequences (e.g., excessive spending, increased sexual activity)

- Hallucinating or having delusions, which can result from severe episodes of mania

Lows (Depression)

- Feeling extremely sad or hopeless

- Being in an irritable mood

- Having no desire for once enjoyable activities

- Loss of interest in life

- Sleeping too much or having trouble sleeping

- Showing changes in appetite or weight

- Having little or no energy or moving slowly

- Difficulty concentrating, paying attention and remembering things

- Feeling aches and pains for no reason

- Problems with work, social or family life

- Finding minor decisions overwhelming

- Obsessing over feelings of loss, personal failure, guilt or helplessness

- Having recurrent thoughts or talk of death or suicide.

- Feeling worthless or guilty

An organisation in Australia called "Headspace" is the National Youth Mental Health Foundation which provides early intervention mental health services to 12-25 year olds. On their website they quote the following statistics based on their research concerning bipolar disorder.[4]

- At least one in every 100 people will experience bipolar disorder at some time during their lives.

- In Australia, it is estimated that approximately 1.8% of males and 1.7% of females have had bipolar disorder in the previous 12 months.

- In young Australians aged 16-24 years, it is estimated that approximately 3.2% of males and 3.6% of females have had bipolar disorder in their lifetime.

- Bipolar disorder is the ninth leading contributor to the burden of disease and injury in Australian females aged 15-24 years and the tenth leading contributor for males of the same age.

- Overall, about 50% of people who develop bipolar disorder will do so by the time they are in their early to mid 20s.

4 http://headspace.org.au/health-professionals/bipolar-disorders/

- Bipolar disorder in young people may sometimes be misdiagnosed as depression.

- Australian researchers have found that from the average age of symptom onset (17.5 years), there was a delay of approximately 12.5 years before a diagnosis of bipolar disorder was made.

The prevalence of bipolar disorder is probably higher than the statistics suggest as many cases are often undetected or misdiagnosed.

Generally, in order to be diagnosed with bipolar a person must have experienced major depression (a severe and intense depression) that was present for at least two weeks. Then, they must have manifested at least four of the following symptoms of mania:

- Need little sleep

- Talk extremely fast

- Have racing thoughts

- Easily distracted so their attention keeps shifting from one topic to the next

- Feel extremely powerful, important or great

- Engage in reckless behaviour with money, sex or business deals

From associating with other sufferers of bipolar and from our own personal experience we have discovered that, when someone is manic, they typically deny that they have a problem and get angry if you suggest that they do. In the early days of Jenny's beginning to have manic episodes, I (Robert) would point out what I was seeing and because Jenny was feeling so good, she would often become defensive at any suggestion she was becoming manic. We think the reason for this is because for the sufferer of bipolar there is such a strong desire to feel 'normal' and not depressed, that any hint of change is a hope that normalcy has arrived. Then to be told that it is only a fleeting transition into a state of mania causes a sense of frustration and at times anger.

Bipolar is generally divided into two classifications[5] as follows:

- **Bipolar 1 disorder** is when the person experiences oscillating hyper manic (extreme 'highs', often with psychotic features) and depressive episodes. The severity and duration of these episodes often lasts at least seven days and may result in hospitalisation.

- **Bipolar 2 disorder** is when the person experiences depressive episodes shifting back and forth with a milder form of mania (hypomania) that does not include psychotic features.

At first I (Jenny) didn't know about the classifications of bipolar. As I discovered more about my illness and consulted with my medical and psychiatric doctors I was diagnosed as bipolar 1. For a brief period early on in my illness, I did suffer from occasional psychotic features and hallucinations; however, this has not happened again since the first few years of my illness. My episodes of mania have become more hypomania rather than longer severe hypermania.

From our understanding and research, it appears that the earlier bipolar disorder begins, the more severe the course of the disorder tends to be. In my case, I began experiencing bipolar at the age of twenty-eight and now, twenty-three years later, I have experienced over eighty episodes and at least twenty hospitalisations. The episodes

5 Black Dog Institute give classifications of bipolar on their website
http://www.blackdoginstitute.org.au

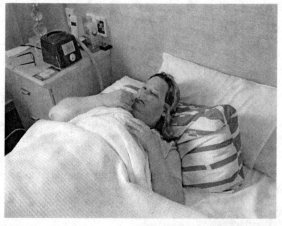

Hospital low

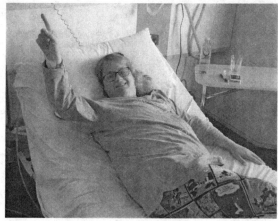

Hospital high

have definitely increased over the last eight years and resulted in most of the stays in hospital.

With the continual advancement in medical science and therapies, there is some good news for sufferers. Today, bipolar disorder is one of the most treatable of mental illnesses and not all people suffering serious mood swings fall into the extreme disturbances of bipolar disorder. Some suffer from cyclothymia disorder causing emotional ups and downs but they're not as extreme as those in bipolar 1 or 2 disorder. With cyclothymia disorder, a person may experience short periods when their mood noticeably shifts up and down from their baseline. It is not as extreme as those who have bipolar disorder and is much less debilitating - not interfering with their ability to function.

Another category of bipolar disorder is called a 'mixed state' and is a combination of manic and depressive symptoms occurring simultaneously. There is estimated at least 40% of people who present with manic symptoms who also have depression symptoms at the same time. The seriousness of the mixed state is that if suicidal thoughts are present in the depression, there may also be sufficient resolve to carry out the act due the mania state. This is why diagnosis and proper treatment are vital.

For some sufferers of chronic bipolar they may be classified as having cyclothymia disorder. This is when the person experiences a chronically unstable mood state for at least two years with mild depression and a milder form of mania that does not include psychotic episodes.

The United States of America broadcaster, CBS, wrote about famous people who have been diagnosed with bipolar in an attempt to highlight the illness and help eliminate the social stigma.

> "Many high-profile successful people, including Demi Lovato, Catherine Zeta-Jones and Jean-Claude Van Damme have been diagnosed with bipolar disorder... More than 5 million Americans suffer from the disorder, according to the National Institute of Mental Health. In observance of World Bipolar Day, March 30, 2016, which aimed to raise awareness and eliminate the stigma of the illness, here's a look at famous people with bipolar - many whom became advocates for mental health. Singer Demi Lovato was diagnosed with bipolar disorder when she entered rehab at age 22. Before her

diagnosis she had struggled with bulimia, drug addiction and cutting. She has chosen to use her fame to help eliminate the stigma and advocate for treatment, taking part in a campaign called "Be Vocal: Speak Up for Mental Health" in 2015. Lovato told WomensHealthMag.com she wants women to know that "it's possible to live well, feel well and also find happiness with bipolar disorder or any other mental illness they're struggling with."[6]

Although bipolar disorder causes significant disruption to the life of the sufferer and their family, it is comforting to know that you are not alone in the journey. Many famous people throughout history were thought or retrospectively judged to have had bipolar disorder and remained exceptionally creative and influential leaders. A cursory glance through the internet will provide you with a wide array of people suffering with bipolar including figures like Winston Churchill, Daniel Webster, C.T. Studd, Vincent Van Gogh, Mozart, Beethoven, Mark Twain, Ernest Hemmingway, Hans Christian Anderson and many more.

We believe that the diagnosis of bipolar disorder is the first step to developing a plan that may help save your life, uplift your soul and rescue you from the confusion and despair of this debilitating disorder. If you suspect you have the illness consult a doctor, psychologist or psychiatrist as soon as you can. If someone you know is suffering from this disorder, please be patient with them and help them find help.

---

6 http://www.cbsnews.com/pictures/famous-people-celebrities-bipolar/

CHAPTER 4

THINGS THAT ARE BROKEN
DON'T WORK RIGHT

DISORDER

We live in what theologians call 'a fallen world' following the sin of Adam and Eve in the garden of Eden. This is what is referred to as the 'fall of man', and we are living in a post-Eden world subjected to the curse of sin.

The apostle Paul summed up the results of the sin of Adam in a few verses when writing to the church at Rome. He reminded us that sin entered this world through the actions of Adam and all the sicknesses and illnesses that now happen in this world are a consequence of sin entering in. "*Wherefore, as by one man sin entered into the world, and death by sin; and so death passed upon all men, for that all have sinned:*" (*Romans 5:12*)

Prior to the fall of man, there was no sickness, no suffering and no mental illness. Similarly, the Bible tells us of a time in the future when God will create a new heaven and new earth where there will be no more sin. "*And I saw a new heaven and a new earth: for the first heaven and the first earth were passed away; and there was no more sea. And I John saw the holy city, new Jerusalem, coming down from God out of heaven, prepared as a bride adorned for her husband. And I heard a great voice out of heaven saying, Behold, the tabernacle of God is with men, and he will dwell with them, and they shall be his people, and God himself shall be with them, and be their God. And God shall wipe away all tears from their eyes; and there shall be no more death, neither sorrow, nor crying, neither shall there be any more pain: for the former things are passed away." (Revelation 21:1-4)*

The songwriter of old, Sanford Fillmore Bennett, wrote a great hymn describing the bliss and rest of heaven. The song is called "In the Sweet By and By." But for the time being, we live in the "Nasty Now and Now" enduring the infirmities and afflictions of this life.

From a Christian standpoint, it is useful to know what part of you is affected by bipolar and how it is affected.

Many people far more qualified than we are have written on the medical aspects of bipolar disorder. Since neither of us are medical professionals or trained in the field of mental health, we do not for one moment think we have the intricate medical and psychiatric knowledge to define bipolar disorder and its effects in medical terms. Our description of this illness has been gleaned from the many valuable public resources available on the subject - published by reputable doctors and medical institutions, together with our own personal experiences. Accordingly, the information that is included in this chapter is based on our own personal research, experience and understanding. By no means do we consider ourselves medical experts and if you desire more specific information on bipolar, we suggest you talk with the medical professionals in your life and research reliable medical sources.

However, from a spiritual aspect, we both believe the Bible provides many answers to questions often asked about mankind and what it is that makes us who we are.

According to the Bible, mankind is distinct from the rest of creation, including the animals, in that we are made in the image of God who is a tripartite God - Father, Son and Holy Spirit. God is one, yet three. So too the Bible defines all human beings as having three parts – spirit, soul and body. In writing to the church at Thessalonica, the apostle Paul reminds us of God's plan for our whole being – *"And the very God of peace sanctify you wholly; and I pray God your whole **spirit** and **soul** and **body** be preserved blameless unto the coming of our Lord Jesus Christ."* (1 Thessalonians 5:23)

Those who believe this are called "trichotomists" and believe man is a tripartite being made in the image of a triune God. Notice the use of plural pronouns in the Scripture describing the creation of man and woman. *"And God said, Let **us** make man in **our** image, after **our** likeness: and let them have dominion over the fish of the sea, and over the fowl of the air, and over the cattle, and over all the earth, and over every creeping thing that creepeth upon the earth. So God created man in his own image, in the image of God created he him; male and female created he them."* (Genesis 1:26-27)

What does God look like? What is the image of God? Has anyone ever seen God in the flesh? These questions were answered when God became flesh and dwelt as a man in the form of the Lord Jesus Christ. *"No man hath seen God at any time; the only begotten Son, which is in the bosom of the Father, he hath declared him."* (John 1:18).

One of Jesus' disciples asked to see God the Father and Jesus told Him that by seeing Him (Jesus) he was seeing the Father because they are one. *"Philip saith unto him, Lord, shew us the Father, and it sufficeth us. Jesus saith unto him, Have I been so long time with you, and yet hast thou not known me, Philip? he that hath seen me hath seen the Father; and how sayest thou then, Shew us the Father? Believest thou not that I am in the Father, and the Father in me? the words that I speak unto you I speak not of myself: but the Father that dwelleth in me, he doeth the works. Believe me that I am in the Father, and the Father in me: or else believe me for the very works' sake." (John 14:8-11)*

In describing the Lord Jesus, the Bible says He is the express image of God and is the fullness of the Godhead in a body. *"For in him dwelleth all the fulness of the Godhead bodily." (Colossians 2:9)*

The Bible describes Jesus as the Son of God having a body, soul and a spirit. So, if we are made in the image of God, then we too have these three parts to us, as the scriptures teach us.

Created in the image of God, man is likewise a trinity. He has a spiritual nature that is separate and distinct from the body in which it dwells. The body is made up of physical material that can be seen and touched. But, the soul and the spirit are made up of immaterial aspects, which are intangible. Within the soul and the spirit we have the faculties of intellect, will, emotions, conscience and so forth which make up our personality. These immaterial characteristics exist beyond the physical lifespan of the human body and are therefore eternal. The body is the physical container that houses the soul and spirit on this earth.

Knowing we have a body, soul and spirit, we can then determine how bipolar disorder impacts the whole person and then look at various options and ways in which we can manage the illness both physically and spiritually.

Firstly, we will discuss the body.

THE HUMAN BODY AND BIPOLAR

As humans we have a physical body which is incredibly complex and yet perfectly designed by the Creator God Himself. The Bible records what King David said about our physical being: *"I will praise thee; for I am fearfully and wonderfully made: marvellous are thy works; and that my soul knoweth right well." (Psalm 139:14)*

Throughout the Bible our body is described using various metaphors each reminding us of the temporal and frail nature of the human body. Our body is described as a mere frame made from dust: *"For he knoweth our frame; he remembereth that we are dust." (Psalm 103:14)* Paul describes it like a temporary tent (tabernacle) that will one day be dismantled: *"For we know that if our earthly house of this tabernacle were dissolved, we have a building of God, an house not made with hands, eternal in the heavens." (2 Corinthians 5:1)*

In comparing the spiritual and physical aspects of a human, the Bible refers to the body as the 'outward man' that is perishing. *"For which cause we faint not; but though our outward man perish, yet the inward man is renewed day by day." (2 Corinthians 4:16)*

The mortal body is compared to a house of clay that is so easily destroyed in comparison to an immortal God. *"Shall mortal man be more just than God? shall a man be more pure than his maker? Behold, he put no trust in his servants; and his angels he charged with folly: How much less in them that dwell in houses of clay, whose foundation is in the dust, which are crushed before the moth? They are destroyed from morning to evening: they perish for ever without any regarding it." (Job 4:17-20)*

What these verses teach us is that our bodies will dissolve and perish. Our human bodies are subject to the effects of the fall of man and will get sick, wear out and eventually stop living. We are physically fragile, mortal and temporal. This is why we are susceptible to diseases, sicknesses, genetic and chromosome deficiencies, chemical imbalances and a host of other issues that can plague our bodies. This accounts for the pain we suffer in our bodies. For women, the Bible describes the pain of childbearing as a consequence of the sin of Eve. After the fall of man, our bodies are greatly affected by the curse upon the earth and mankind. *"Unto the woman he said, I will greatly multiply thy sorrow and thy conception; in sorrow thou shalt bring forth children; and thy desire shall be to thy husband, and he shall rule over thee. And unto Adam he said, Because thou hast hearkened unto the voice of thy wife, and hast eaten of the tree, of which I commanded thee, saying, Thou shalt not eat of it: cursed is the ground for thy sake; in sorrow shalt thou eat of it all the days of thy life; Thorns also and thistles shall it bring forth to thee; and thou shalt eat the herb of the field; In the sweat of thy face shalt thou eat bread, till thou return unto the ground; for out of it wast thou taken: for dust thou art, and unto dust shalt thou return."* (Genesis 3:16-19)

The body gives us mobility and through its five senses, it makes us conscious of the world in which we live. The body houses all of the organs which work the circulatory system, the nervous system, the muscular system, the digestive system and many other incredibly designed systems that make our bodies work.

When it comes to bipolar, the parts of the body mainly affected are the brain and the nervous system.

Secondly, we will discuss the soul.

THE HUMAN SOUL AND BIPOLAR DISORDER

The word 'soul' in the Bible comes from the Greek word in the New Testament called 'psyche.' In the Old Testament the Hebrew word is 'nephesh.'

We see the use of the word 'psyche' in psychology and psychiatry.

The soul consists of the mind (which includes the conscience), the will and the emotions. The soul and the spirit are mysteriously tied together and make up what the scriptures call the 'heart.'

The soul is the seat of the emotions, affections, desires and provides us with self-consciousness. We have the ability to know and feel through the soul. The soul is the real you; it is the 'inner man.'

The Lord Jesus spoke of His soul having emotions:-

His soul was sorrowful - *"Then saith he unto them, My soul is exceeding sorrowful, even unto death: tarry ye here, and watch with me." (Matthew 26:38)*

His soul was troubled - *"Now is my soul troubled; and what shall I say? Father, save me from this hour: but for this cause came I unto this hour." (John 12:27)*

The soul of man is the part that will live forever. In comparing the temporal nature of the body and the eternal nature of the soul, Jesus gave a very stern warning to all of mankind to ensure they turn to God as a believer. *"And fear not them which kill the body, but are not able to kill the soul: but rather fear him which is able to destroy both soul and body in hell." (Matthew 10:28)*

Whilst medicines, vitamins and supplements can definitely help with the chemical imbalances and mineral deficiencies in our brains and bodies, it is the soul of man that also needs to be addressed in terms of thinking, feeling and decision making.

Many of the mental battles are not always happening in the brain (the physical organ) but they happen within the soul and spirit of man, within the intellect, emotions, will, conscience and heart. We must always make a clear distinction between the brain (physical) and the mind (spiritual).

Whilst there are many helpful secular psychological strategies available to assist sufferers of bipolar to manage and deal with their illness, we feel God and His Word provide immense help to speak to the soul which He created.

The Bible states the place in which we do battle is in the soul of man – especially in the mind. The apostle Peter tells us the war of lusts and desires take place in the soul, our intellect, emotions and will. *"Dearly beloved, I beseech you as strangers and pilgrims, abstain from fleshly lusts, which **war against the soul**;" (1 Peter 2:11)*

In the Bible, the apostle Paul wrote about the struggles we have in our thinking and also likens it to a war, *"But I see another law in my members (body including your brain) **warring against** the law of **my mind**, and bringing me into captivity to the law of sin which is in my members (body)." (Romans 7:23)* (emphasis added)

God inspired Peter to write to let us know about the impact that external stimulus can have not just upon the body, but upon the soul (mind, heart and will). Also God can help a person be delivered from the negative aspects that can affect the soul. *"And delivered just Lot, vexed with the filthy conversation of the wicked: (For that righteous man dwelling among them, in seeing and hearing, vexed his righteous soul from day to day with their unlawful deeds;) The Lord knoweth how to deliver the godly out of temptations, and to reserve the unjust unto the day of judgment to be punished:" (2 Peter 2:7-9)*

This is why we firmly believe in the power of God's Word to help anyone with matters that affect their soul. The Word of God can aid, assist, provide answers, renew our thinking and at times even allow sufferers from mental illness to find healing through God. *"Wherefore lay apart all filthiness and superfluity of naughtiness, and receive with meekness the engrafted word, which is able to save your souls." (James 1:21)*

It is with the Word of God and the Holy Spirit that our minds can be renewed daily to help manage and correct the negative thought patterns and wrong thinking that so often plague sufferers with bipolar disorder. *"I beseech you therefore, brethren, by the mercies of God, that ye present your bodies a living sacrifice, holy, acceptable unto God, which is your reasonable service. And be not conformed to this world: but be ye transformed **by the renewing of your mind**, that ye may prove what is that good, and acceptable, and perfect, will of God." (Romans 12:1-2)*

Finally, we have the third part of mankind, the spirit.

THE HUMAN SPIRIT AND BIPOLAR DISORDER

In the New Testament the word 'spirit' is translated from the Greek word 'pneuma' and from the Hebrew word 'ruach' when found in the Old Testament.

'Pneuma' means air or life force. That is why, in the description of the creation of Adam, God breathed life into Adam and he became a living soul. *"And the LORD God formed man of the dust of the ground, and breathed into his nostrils the breath of life; and man became a living soul."* (Genesis 2:7)

Every person has a spirit. The spirit of man is not the individual man or the ego of the man. It is his life source. The soul of man is the real inner you. So, when a person dies, his spirit simply goes back to its maker – God. *"Then shall the dust return to the earth as it was: and the spirit shall return unto God who gave it."* (Ecclesiastes 12:7) What happens to the soul after death is different. Its destiny is determined by whether the person has accepted Jesus Christ as their personal Saviour or not. If a person is saved their soul will go to heaven, but if a person is lost, their soul will go to hell.

The spirit is the part of man that knows. *"For what man knoweth the things of a man, save the spirit of man which is in him? even so the things of God knoweth no man, but the Spirit of God."* (1 Corinthians 2:11)

The spirit in man can be enlightened by God. *"But there is a spirit in man: and the inspiration of the Almighty giveth them understanding."* (Job 32:8)

The spirit of man gives us God-consciousness and when we are born again it gives us the ability to communicate with God. *"The Spirit itself beareth witness with our spirit, that we are the children of God:"* (Romans 8:16) All men have the same spirit. Some men's spirits have been quickened (made alive) when the person was born again. The remainder are still dead in sin.

It is the spirit of man that must be born again by believing in and receiving Jesus Christ as Saviour. Thus the spirit is quickened and made alive giving man God-consciousness, the ability to commune freely with God. *"Jesus answered, Verily, verily, I say unto thee, Except a man be born of water and of the Spirit, he cannot enter into the kingdom of God. That which is born of the flesh is flesh; and that which is born of the Spirit is spirit. Marvel not that I said unto thee, Ye must be born again." (John 3:5-7)*

In the scriptures, the spiritual part of our soul and our spirit are often spoken of as working together, yet the Lord clearly speaks of them separately. The Bible says God actually divides the soul and spirit through the work of the Word of God. It pierces our heart to discern our thoughts and intents. God does this work in our spiritual being and convicts us, comforts us and challenges us through His Word in the process - something that only God can do. *"For the word of God is quick, and powerful, and sharper than any two edged sword, piercing even to the dividing asunder of soul and spirit, and of the joints and marrow (body), and is a discerner of the thoughts and intents of the heart." (Hebrews 4:12)* (The word *'body'* has been added for emphasis only)

In summary, our whole being is affected by bipolar disorder and needs to be considered in the treatment and management of the illness.

We do not have clear understanding of precisely what causes bipolar disorder, yet we do know from a spiritual perspective. All human problems ultimately stem from the disobedience of Adam and Eve, which brought sin and evil into society and into individual's lives, but there does not appear to be any particular sin problem in the lives of most people suffering from bipolar disorder. Many fine Christians struggle for much of their lives with this distressing difficulty.

Within the complexity of the soul and spirit of mankind, there possibly are some physiological factors, as well as long-standing emotional conflicts that can contribute to bipolar disorder or at least form the basis of triggers that can bring about an episode or the onset of the illness.

However, clearly there do appear to be physical links to possible causes. In fact, the higher frequency of bipolar disorder among first-degree relatives strongly suggests a genetic basis as *a* major, if not *the* major, factor in causing the disorder. Whilst genes are involved in bipolar disorder, it isn't clear how or to what extent. Hopefully, genetic research will someday provide significant advances in stabilising or even curing this devastating illness. Psychiatrists Dinah Miller, Annette Hanson and Steven Roy Davis wrote the following:

> "We have reasons for believing that psychiatric disorders must certainly be mediated by biological factors. For one thing, psychiatric illnesses run in families, even when family members are separated at birth. Research has shown that genetic links and even specific genes, may be associated with different disorders. Many studies have shown that the biological features of groups of people with illnesses are different from those same features in groups of people without those illnesses. What we don't have, yet, is a specific reliable test for a certain genotype or enzyme level, or a brain scan finding that indicates that a specific person has a specific disease. If a person goes to the doctor because of increased thirst or urination and has a lab test done and it shows markedly elevated blood sugar levels, then that patient most certainly has diabetes. But with a few rare exceptions, such as Huntington's disease or Jacob-Creutzfelt dementia, there's nothing like this in psychiatry — no blood

test, no x-ray, no CT scan that yields a definitive diagnosis. In psychiatry, blood tests are ordered to rule out medical conditions that masquerade as psychiatric illnesses — especially thyroid conditions or high ammonia levels — or to monitor medication levels to make sure medications are not damaging a patient's organs."[7]

However, we now have enough medical research plus volumes of psychiatric case-studies to show that the body, the physical aspects of the illness, are real and not just 'all in the head'.

Over the past decade, due to research findings in the connection of mental illness to biology, the struggle for recognition of the disorder as organic and real has strengthened and helped in the removal of stigmatisation. Now sufferers from bipolar disorder know that their illness has a physiological basis.

Whilst there is still no test available that can prove a chemical imbalance directly causes this disorder, there is a common agreement amongst the medical profession that much of the bipolar disorder is brought about by deficiencies in serotonin levels in the brain. Chemicals like serotonin (neurotransmitters) aid in the communication of information between neurons in the brain. The chemicals move across a small gap (synapse) from one neuron, where they may be accepted by the next neuron, at a specialised site called a receptor. In laymen's terms, it is thought that if there is a serotonin deficiency then the neurons don't 'fire' effectively, potentially leading to a bipolar episode. There are many types of chemicals that act as neurotransmitter substances, some of them include: Acetylcholine (ACh), Dopamine (DA), Norepinephrine (NE), Serotonin (5-HT), Histamine and Epinephrine.

---

7 http://www.peteearley.com/2015/01/30/mental-illnesses-caused-chemical-imbalances/

Research has identified areas of brain activity that indicate a causal relationship to the symptoms of bipolar. It is thought that the brain activity could be a *result* of the disorder rather than a *cause*. Further studies have shown the PET brain scan differences in blood flow to the frontal cortex showing a sharp decrease in activity in the brain of a depressed person compared to others who are not depressed.[8] These scientific discoveries have now helped the medical profession recognise that sufferers of bipolar potentially have physical deficiencies that may be attributing to the cause of the illness.

"There appear to be consistent findings in the neuroimaging literature that suggest an etiological model for bipolar disorder that involves abnormalities in the structure and function of the amygdala, but also depends on the failure of prefrontal cortical regions to modulate amygdala activity."[9]

"There is increasing attention being paid to the brain regions that are dysfunctional in bipolar disorder - bipolar disorder both in children and in adults. It appears that one important region is the amygdala, which is a little area in our brain; 'amygdala' means 'almond' in Greek. It's inside our temporal lobes so the amygdala is located in the brain, and it is important in terms of identifying in the environment what's important to us emotionally. If we see danger for example, the amygdala will become activated. If we see anything that we consider to be very rewarding, the amygdala will become activated. There is some evidence in both adults and children with bipolar disorder that the amygdala tends to respond more in people with bipolar disorder than it does in people without bipolar disorder, so that maybe the brains of people

8 PET scans can be viewed on the internet on many websites. See *http://psychyogi.org/depression/*
9 https://www.ncbi.nlm.nih.gov/pubmed/18838042

with bipolar disorder are seeing the world as more emotional than are people without bipolar disorder. There is also evidence in children with bipolar disorder that the amygdala is smaller than it should be. Other parts of the brain that people have been very interested in bipolar disorder include the prefrontal cortex. The prefrontal cortex has many different parts but the two parts of interest are the so called dorsal lateral prefrontal cortex and the ventral prefrontal cortex. The ventral prefrontal cortex is very tightly connected to the amygdala, and like the amygdala deals with what's rewarding and what isn't rewarding in our environment. There is some literature and some data that like the amygdala, the ventral lateral prefrontal cortex may be too active at times in people with bipolar disorder. On the other hand the dorsolateral prefrontal cortex is the part that's kind of the rational part; it's the part that figures out what's going on in the world and figures out how can we best strategize to get what we want. There's some evidence that that's less active in people with bipolar disorder than in people without. So putting it all together, you've kind of got a situation where the emotional parts of the brain may be particularly active in people with bipolar disorder, and the part of the brain that supposed to sort of damp down the emotional parts of the brain may be a bit less active in people with bipolar disorder."[10]

This news has been a strange source of comfort for me (Jenny). It has helped me to know that my illness is not just a figment of my imagination, but rather it is part of my physiology.

While we can just focus on and treat the physical aspects of the illness, we believe it is in the spiritual areas of our lives where we

10 Doctor Ellen Leibenluft discusses brain regions associated with bipolar disorder - https://www.dnalc.org/view/2355-neuropathology-of-bipolar-disorder.html

can be better equipped to deal with and manage the effects that bipolar disorder has on the physical, bodily parts, both externally and internally. By understanding we have three parts to our being and addressing the needs of the soul and the spirit as well, we seek to treat the whole person.

Because God is the maker of us all, He knows best what we need to renew our minds and align our thinking to handle the onslaughts and attacks that come because of the physical illness in the body and brain. Further along in this book we will discuss how God's Word has helped shape and change our thinking over the course of our bipolar journey.

CHAPTER 5

DEALING WITH STIGMA

DENIAL

Most people live a fairly normal, balanced mental health life, so they have no idea what it is like to be a person living with a mental illness. They just label me (Jenny) 'crazy'. Then add Christianity into the mix and amongst some Christian circles I am labelled a 'sinner' who needs to get right with God so that I can be healed of my sickness or delivered from my demons. Because, real Christians don't suffer from a mental illness – or do they?

To further polarise the beliefs on mental illness, famous celebrities often throw their unfounded opinions into the mix. In 2005, actor Tom Cruise, who has been an adherent of Scientology for nearly two decades, claimed that anti-depressants are 'dangerous' and that mental health care is 'pseudo-science'. Mr. Cruise asserted that exercise and vitamins successfully treat depression, despite the convincing and conclusive evidence to the contrary. What Mr. Cruise did not mention is that Scientology Inc. teaches as a 'scientific fact' that aliens from outer space created the entire mental health care profession on Earth in order to enslave humanity. In a taped lecture by Scientology Inc.'s creator, L. Ron Hubbard, Mr. Hubbard insisted that space alien psychiatrists created pain, sex and death and that modern mental health care professionals are controlled and manipulated by these space aliens. Interestingly, in 1947, during his first divorce, Hubbard was diagnosed as schizophrenic and begged the United States Veterans Administration for psychiatric treatment.[11]

The reality is, bipolar disorder is a mental illness. Mental illnesses in general are often disputed in many Christian circles and not readily accepted, being seen as a 'hidden disability'.

Because some of the psychotic symptoms that can be manifested with bipolar – such as delusional thinking, paranoia and at times hallucinations, especially in manic episodes with lack of sleep - the accusation of demonic possession is made. In some churches the person will be subjected to attempts to cast out the evil spirits.

Some people believe that bipolar disorder and other mental health problems are only symptomatic of, or consequences of, demonic possession. They believe the sufferer needs to be truly born again to be cured of the illness through prayer and faith.

Some people also believe that, for a Christian to resort to the fields of psychiatry and psychiatric drugs, he or she is dabbling in crafts that have their origins in Satan, not in God, and must be totally rejected.

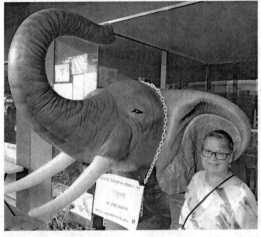

These deeply-held beliefs are not easily changed and the stigmas become entrenched. Most of the stigma associated with bipolar disorder is based on a lack of information and understanding about

11 http://www.schizophrenia.com/sznews/archives/002374.html#

the illness. Being well informed about bipolar can help to recognise some of the misconceptions involved with the disorder.

All I (Jenny) can do is to tell my own story with lived experiences and Biblical beliefs, to help break down the stigma of mental illness in our society and especially in our churches. I believe it is time to start talking about mental health. With one in five Australians experiencing symptoms of mental illness each year, it's time that mental health stops being the elephant in the room. It's my heart's desire to give bipolar a voice and help towards breaking the silence and stigma surrounding this illness.

It is easy to understand why some Christians do hold to the position that real Christians don't suffer from mental illness and any who do are stigmatised in a negative way within society and in the church.

The word 'lunatic' occurs twice in the Bible. One is in reference to people who were brought to Jesus for healing and one concerns a young boy whose behaviour labelled him such.

> *"Lord, have mercy on my son: for he is **lunatick**, and sore vexed: for ofttimes he falleth into the fire, and oft into the water. And I brought him to thy disciples, and they could not cure him. Then Jesus answered and said, O faithless and perverse generation, how long shall I be with you? how long shall I suffer you? bring him hither to me. And Jesus rebuked the **devil**; and he departed out of him: and the child was cured from that very hour." (Matthew 17:15-18)*

There is also the account of a man living among the tombs who was cutting himself and had seemingly supernatural strength. He was a demon-possessed man whom Jesus healed and cast the demons out into a herd of pigs which subsequently ran over a hill and plunged into the sea and drowned.

"And they came over unto the other side of the sea, into the country of the Gadarenes. And when he was come out of the ship, immediately there met him out of the tombs a man with an **unclean spirit**, Who had his dwelling among the tombs; and no man could bind him, no, not with chains: Because that he had been often bound with fetters and chains, and the chains had been plucked asunder by him, and the fetters broken in pieces: neither could any man tame him. And always, night and day, he was in the mountains, and in the tombs, crying, and cutting himself with stones. But when he saw Jesus afar off, he ran and worshipped him, And cried with a loud voice, and said, What have I to do with thee, Jesus, thou Son of the most high God? I adjure thee by God, that thou torment me not. For he said unto him, Come out of the man, thou **unclean spirit**. And he asked him, What is thy name? And he answered, saying, My name is Legion: for we are many. And he besought him much that he would not send them away out of the country. Now there was there nigh unto the mountains a great herd of swine feeding. And all the **devils** besought him, saying, Send us into the swine, that we may enter into them. And forthwith Jesus gave them leave. And the **unclean spirits** went out, and entered into the swine: and the herd ran violently down a steep place into the sea, (they were about two thousand;) and were choked in the sea. And they that fed the swine fled, and told it in the city, and in the country. And they went out to see what it was that was done. And they come to Jesus, and see him that was possessed with the **devil**, and had the legion, sitting, and clothed, and in his **right mind**: and they were afraid." (Mark 5:1-15)

In both of these accounts the cause of the mental afflictions was demonic. This is one of the main reasons why people believe mental illness is connected to satanic strongholds. It is further not uncommon for people suffering with mental illness to also manifest religious mania in their beliefs and words.

Whilst demonic oppression and possession can certainly be a factor in some cases of mental illness, as with many other ailments, it is very unwise to naively label every cause of a mental health problem the result of a devil or unclean spirit. (We will discuss this issue in more detail in the next chapter.)

It is often that which we don't understand, that we fear. Fear of the unknown causes of mental illness makes it an easy target to simply attribute a spiritual reason to the illness. However this quick spiritual diagnosis can be devastating and dangerous. Many people in their distress and torment of mind will come to their church seeking help and deliverance from their affliction. So to be told this is only a spiritual issue, they may end up, as many do, feeling like an inadequate Christian who doesn't pray enough, read the Bible enough, fast enough or do enough of the many other spiritual practices. This can leave a Christian feeling very stigmatised and without hope, often being relegated to the place of a second-rate Christian, or not even a Christian at all!

I (Jenny) have spoken to some people who have been told by church leaders that their bipolar disorder is not a valid illness and the sufferer is blatantly accused of 'making it up,' leaving them confused after being diagnosed with certainty by their doctor or psychiatrist.

It is ironic that nobody generally questions a person who has a heart condition or a broken leg suggesting they have a demonic issue that has caused the problem. However, the moment you bring the illness back to something that is difficult to scientifically test and see - like a mental illness in the brain - you are under spiritual scrutiny.

Sadly, if it is ever known in the church that an individual has bipolar disorder, that person may feel the ugliness of stigma that surrounds anything people fear or do not understand. Nobody should be shunned or even asked to leave a church simply because people are afraid and ignorant of bipolar or any other mental illness.

Bipolar disorder is a health condition like diabetes and not a personality flaw. While certain illness-related behaviours might be socially unacceptable, these behaviours are symptoms of a treatable illness.

Sometimes the person's own stigma about mental illness can cause them to lose confidence and belief that any change is possible. Lack of confidence might prevent them from pursuing manageable opportunities and goals that could enrich their lives. This is why we need to not live in denial but rather speak out about the reality and the help that is available for bipolar sufferers.

After preaching at a church on one occasion, I (Robert) recall being told, "You are very brave to come out and talk publicly about your wife's illness." I was asked, "Aren't you concerned about how people in the church will view you and your wife in ministry now knowing she has bipolar?" At first I was shocked and began to question my transparency from the pulpit, but this feeling was soon nullified as many more people came and thanked me for being open and honest and began to tell of their own stories.

Over the years, even concerned friends and fellow church members have asked me (Jenny) questions like, "Are you sure that you have bipolar disorder?" or "Could it just be you've had too much on your plate being a pastor's wife?" Some have suggested, "Maybe you should pray about it and just trust God." All of these well-meaning questions and suggestions often left me further stigmatised, and questioning my own diagnosis and even my faith.

You start to wonder, "I love the Lord and I think I am trying my best to live a good Christian life, so why hasn't God healed my bipolar disorder?" I am sure from my conversations with other Christians who suffer from bipolar or depression that such questioning and introspection causes further confusion on the part of the individual with bipolar disorder and has even turned some away from Christianity entirely.

The following story is an account of a Christian woman who suffered the stigmatisation that often accompanies mental illness:

> "You can't judge a book by its cover—nor can you tell what's inside someone by his or her outside appearance. If you could see me, you'd agree that my appearance is fairly ordinary. I've been married for eighteen years, about one or two of which could be described by the word normal—at least as the world defines that concept. As the medical world defines things, I am mentally ill. By the time such an official diagnosis could be made, it was actually something of a relief. Does that statement shock you? You see, I'd been told I had demons inside of me. A formal medical diagnosis was very helpful; it made it possible for me to be treated properly and to better understand the many facets of my condition. I was hospitalised for many years. That period is over, but even now I must spend time in hospitals when I face a crisis. Sometimes people want to know how I can be a Christian and still have these conditions, particularly conditions that could lead people like me to harm themselves. But they don't

understand the reality of depression as I do. I feel better about all of it when I think about people of great faith who faced depression like mine—people such as Jeremiah, David and Elijah. There were times in our country when people like me would have been put away somewhere, out of sight and out of mind. But we've made progress since then and I can find freedom in talking about my depression and even reaching out to others who are coping with what I've been through. On my good days, you're likely to find me chatty, loving, caring and serving others. I can take responsibility for myself. I pray, read the Bible and try to work through the darker memories from my past. On my bad days, I can simply be thankful for those loving people who care enough to reach out to me. My world becomes black and unmanageable and I become unwilling to look in the mirror or eat. I spend my time terrified, crying, hearing voices that I know aren't there and longing to lose myself in the darkness or to embrace the final release of death. I have days when I get lost and can't find my way home. This often makes me afraid to go out the front door or into the backyard. I have other days when I weep for hours for no apparent reason. Sometimes the stimulus of the world is so overwhelming that I can't cope and my only response is either to flee to the safety of a stronger individual or simply to the comfort of darkness. Those are simply the everyday details of life when you cope with depression. For me to function on a daily basis, I need the help of my husband, my Christian therapist, my psychiatrist, my close friends, my medication and my Lord Jesus. That's the nature of the life I live. And yet, I must tell you that even on my darkest days - even when life is a deep tunnel with no light visible to me - I can still say I've seen Jesus. I've seen Him with the eyes of my spirit, even if the eyes of my mind and heart are blinded. I can feel His presence, even if I can't feel anything else but pain and panic. I'm so grateful that He is my Saviour, for without Him, I'm very certain I would be dead."[12]

As Christians, we look to our pastors and teachers for Godly advice and counsel and place a measure of trust in their spiritual leadership and discernment. For this reason alone, I believe religious leaders should never advise a dutiful Christian to stop taking their medication, assuring them, "God will heal you." For many sufferers of mental illness and bipolar in particular, if they suddenly go off their medication they stand a good chance of plummeting into a bipolar episode to one or both extremes. For some people this may even trigger self-harm or suicidal thoughts. This is a matter of life and death and in my opinion and experience should not be treated lightly by spiritual leaders.

As a Christian with bipolar, I (Jenny) believe my illness does have a chemical biological basis and although it has spiritual dimensions, it is not the work of the devil that has given me bipolar disorder. However, I am not ignorant of Satan's wiles and devices and know he can work through my illness by creating temptations for me to give up and give in to wrong thought patterns.

For example, there have been times where I allowed the sin of pride to pull me down by yielding to temptation to think I don't need any medication and could manage my illness by myself. Yes, there were times when I was able to come off medication under medical supervision, but then there were times I took myself off medication because I started to think I knew better than the doctors and didn't want to be stigmatised any more. I realised it was my pride that made

---

12 Testimony from a family friend of David Jeremiah from his book "A Bend in the Road" Page 80, 2000, W Publishing Group, Nashville Tennessee

it hard for me to accept my illness and at times I was really bitter at God for what was happening.

Other times I have yielded to the temptation to use my sickness as an excuse for laziness and to let everyone take over my responsibilities in life. The few times I did this, I knew I was just frustrated with how I was feeling and felt nobody really understood, and it was a way of getting a weird kind of revenge on others. But once again, the deceitfulness of sin and the flesh always have a way of coming back to hurt you. I do not think it is helpful for those who suffer from bipolar disorder to use it as an excuse for why they are the way they are or do what they do. I think we need to take responsibility and not blame our disorder.

Over time, I have learned to spot these temptations and resist them with the truths of God's Word, prayer and the counsel of my husband and doctors.

On that note, I thank God for the wonderful doctors He has brought into my life, from the early years with Dr David Robinson and then to Dr Mary Russell for many years. For the last several years I have been privileged to be under the care of psychiatrist Dr Lynne Steele and my family doctor who has always encouraged me as a Christian to trust in the Lord, Dr Sandy Prasad. I truly believe that God has worked through the doctors and the medications, and they should be embraced by sufferers of mental illness as a vital part to their well-being.

As Christians, we believe everything that happens in our life is 'Father Filtered' and we should always pray and seek the Lord's advice on all matters in our life, especially our health. He made us and knows us and it is unwise to just seek the advice of doctors. You must seek the Lord that He may direct you to the right doctor or treatment that you need. Whatever you do, make sure you seek the Lord. Don't be like King Asa in the Bible who neglected the Lord. Who knows if he would have lived longer? *"And Asa in the thirty and ninth year of his reign was diseased in his feet, until his disease was exceeding great: yet in his disease he sought not to the LORD, but to the physicians."* *(2 Chronicles 16:12)*

These are just some of the issues that people with bipolar disorder must grapple with if they are Christians. The stigma of being a Christian with a mental illness needs to be broken and we are thankful that more and more Christian leaders are speaking out about the subject; some making bold confessions of their own struggles with mental health issues.

If you have negative beliefs about bipolar and other mental illnesses, be careful not to pass these on to a person suffering from a mental illness. It is not helpful. In fact, it can dramatically impact a sufferer and may even trigger further episodes if they are confronted in a vulnerable moment. Remember, living a better life is a meaningful goal for all of us, whatever our circumstances and experiences. But if you suffer from severe mental illness, like bipolar disorder, a better life can seem out of reach. Healing and help for bipolar sufferers is about not being stigmatised, socially isolated and lonely. It's about having friends, someone to love, something to do, something to be part of and something to look forward to. The focus has to be on supporting recovery, spiritual encouragement, enabling mental well-being as well as building networks of support. It's time to break the silence and stigma surrounding mental health issues.

"There is a particular kind of pain, elation, loneliness, and terror involved in this kind of madness. When you're high it's tremendous. The ideas and feelings are fast and frequent like shooting stars, and you follow them until you find better and brighter ones. Shyness goes, the right words and gestures are suddenly there, the power to captivate others a felt certainty. There are interests found in uninteresting people. Sensuality is pervasive and the desire to seduce and be seduced irresistible. Feelings of ease, intensity, power, well-being, financial omnipotence, and euphoria pervade one's marrow. But, somewhere, this changes. The fast ideas are far too fast, and there are far too many; overwhelming confusion replaces clarity. Memory goes. Humour and absorption on friends' faces are replaced by fear and concern. Everything previously moving with the grain is now against - - you are irritable, angry, frightened, uncontrollable, and enmeshed totally in the blackest caves of the mind. You never knew those caves were there. It will never end, for madness carves its own reality."*

Kay Redfield Jamison,
An Unquiet Mind: A Memoir of Moods and Madness

CHAPTER 6

THE BIBLE AND BIPOLAR

DOCTRINE

From the beginning of Jesus' public ministry on earth, the gospel writer Matthew tells us of the activities of the Lord. *"And Jesus went about all Galilee, teaching in their synagogues, and preaching the gospel of the kingdom, and healing **all** manner of sickness and **all** manner of disease among the people." (Matthew 4:23)*

The Bible is not a medical encyclopaedia, it doesn't refer to every specific type of illness and disease that was known to be in existence at the time of writing. However, it would be safe to assume that mental illnesses may have been one of the conditions described in the Bible phrase *"all manner of sickness and all manner of disease."*

As a pastor, but even more so, as a husband who has a wife with bipolar, I (Robert) have sought the Scriptures for any passages of the Bible that might relate to the issue of mental illness and especially concerning bipolar disorder.

I have been able to find many verses in the Word of God that speak on the issue of discouragement and depression. However, there is one Bible reference that provides us with an apt description of a person who deals with vacillating between the two poles in life. James, the Lord's half-brother, speaks about being in the state of two minds and wavering back and forth. While this passage is primarily concerned with the lack of wisdom to make consistent and firm decisions and the need for single-minded faith in asking from God, it also gives a metaphor describing the feelings of uncertainty and instability in the mind when a person is double-minded. We can relate the double-mindedness to the two states of thinking between mania and depression. It definitely makes a person *"unstable in ALL his ways."*

> *"If any of you lack wisdom, let him ask of God, that giveth to all men liberally, and upbraideth not; and it shall be given him. But let him ask in faith, nothing wavering. For he that wavereth is like a wave of the sea driven with the wind and tossed. For let not that man think that he shall receive any thing of the Lord. A double minded man is unstable in all his ways."(James 1:5-8)*

Reading these verses, we can visualise the ups and downs in the cycles of the disorder and compare them to the waves of the sea that are *'driven with the wind and tossed.'* How often it has felt like our lives have been *'tossed'* around and all over the place by *'winds'* that are *'driven'* by circumstances of life, genetical makeup and chemical imbalances in the neurotransmitters.

This double-minded thinking leaves the sufferers of bipolar with confusion and instability in their life.

Another Bible character in the Scriptures, Jonah, seems to have displayed some of the symptoms of bipolar episodes. At times he wasn't just sad; he was 'exceedingly' displeased. *"But it displeased Jonah exceedingly, and he was very angry."* (Jonah 4:1) Then within a short period of time he was 'exceedingly' glad. *"And the LORD God prepared a gourd, and made it to come up over Jonah, that it might be a shadow over his head, to deliver him from his grief. So Jonah was exceeding glad of the gourd."* (Jonah 4:6) Finally two verses of Scripture later he wanted to die! *"And it came to pass, when the sun did arise, that God prepared a vehement east wind; and the sun beat upon the head of Jonah, that he fainted, and wished in himself to die, and said, It is better for me to die than to live." (Jonah 4:8)* I'm not saying he was bipolar, but we can definitely relate to the major mood swings!

Throughout the Bible there are other references to individuals living with what would today be described as a mental illness.

It appears that people even in the Old Testament days had some type of understanding of what mental illness was. They may not have understood its causes but they were definitely aware of its manifestation in people's lives. For example, David, in an attempt to avoid trouble, acted as though he had some sort of extreme mental illness and his pretence worked.

> *"And David arose, and fled that day for fear of Saul, and went to Achish the king of Gath. And the servants of Achish said unto him, Is not this David the king of the land? did they not sing one to another of him in dances, saying, Saul hath slain his thousands, and David his ten thousands? And David laid up these words in his heart, and was sore afraid of Achish the king of Gath. And **he changed his behaviour** before them, and **feigned himself mad** in their hands, and scrabbled on the doors of the gate, and let his spittle fall down upon his beard. Then said Achish unto his servants, Lo, ye **see the man is mad**: wherefore then have ye brought him to me? **Have I need of mad men**, that ye have brought this fellow to **play the mad man** in my presence? shall this fellow come into my house?" (1 Samuel 21:10)*

On a side note, it is interesting that once Achish thought David was a '*mad man*' he immediately shunned him and wanted nothing to do with a person who displayed the marks of a certain type of 'abnormal' behaviour. A few thousand years later and there still remains a stigma attached to mental illness.

Another Old Testament incident of mental illness was in the case of the Babylonian king Nebuchadnezzar who actually went insane after being judged by God. He later regained his sanity and praised, extolled and honoured God who is able to humble the proud.

> "*The king spake, and said, Is not this great Babylon, that I have built for the house of the kingdom by the might of my power, and for the honour of my majesty? While the word was in the king's mouth, there fell a voice from heaven, saying, O king Nebuchadnezzar, to thee it is spoken; The kingdom is departed from thee. And they shall drive thee from men, and thy dwelling shall be with the beasts of the field: they shall make thee to eat grass as oxen, and seven times shall pass over thee, until thou know that the most High ruleth in the kingdom of men, and giveth it to whomsoever he will. The same hour was the thing fulfilled upon Nebuchadnezzar: and he was driven from men, and did eat grass as oxen, and his body was wet with the dew of heaven, till his hairs were grown like eagles' feathers, and his nails like birds' claws. And at the end of the days I Nebuchadnezzar lifted up mine eyes unto heaven, and mine understanding returned unto me, and I blessed the most High, and I praised and honoured him that liveth for ever, whose dominion is an everlasting dominion, and his kingdom is from generation to generation: And all the inhabitants of the earth are reputed as nothing: and he doeth according to his will in the army of heaven, and among the inhabitants of the earth:*

and none can stay his hand, or say unto him, What doest thou?
*At the same time **my reason returned unto me**; and for the*
glory of my kingdom, mine honour and brightness returned
unto me; and my counsellors and my lords sought unto me;
and I was established in my kingdom, and excellent majesty
was added unto me. Now I Nebuchadnezzar praise and extol
and honour the King of heaven, all whose works are truth, and
his ways judgment: and those that walk in pride he is able to
abase." (Daniel 4:30-37)

The writer of the book of Proverbs describes a symptom of mania in a person the Bible calls a 'mad man.' This person in a state of mania recklessly shoots flaming arrows in his hyper state of mind. The actions of the mania-driven individual is likened to a person who just shoots his mouth off without caution and later thinks it's alright by claiming it was all a joke; but the damage is done! ***"As a mad man** who casteth firebrands, arrows, and death, So is the man that deceiveth his neighbour, and saith, Am not I in sport?" (Proverbs 26:18)*

On another occasion in the Old Testament a young man was instructed by the prophet, Elisha, to go see a military captain named Jehu and anoint him to be king. He was told by the prophet to call him aside and then pour oil on his head, declare him to be king, then run out of the room! *"Then take the box of oil, and pour it on his head, and say, Thus saith the LORD, I have anointed thee king over Israel. Then open the door, and flee, and tarry not." (2 Kings 9:3)* His bizarre actions earned him the title of being 'mad'. Nobody labelled him as demonic, just crazy! *"Then Jehu came forth to the servants of his lord: and one said unto him, Is all well? wherefore came this **mad fellow** to thee? And he said unto them, Ye know the man, and his communication." (2 Kings 9:11)*

However, in a New Testament account, some accused Jesus of being 'mad' and considered the sign of 'madness' indicated the person had a devil. *"And many of them said, **He hath a devil, and is mad**; why hear ye him?" (John 10:20)*

In another incident in the early church era, the apostle Peter was miraculously released from prison and came to a house where Christians were gathered for prayer. When a young lady named Rhoda heard a knock at the door she went to see who it was. Upon recognising it was Peter she ran to tell the others who assumed she had seen an apparition. She was not regarded as having a devil but simply called 'mad'. *"And they said unto her, **Thou art mad**. But she constantly affirmed that it was even so. Then said they, It is his angel." (Acts 12:15)*

As mentioned in the previous chapter, the lunatic young boy and the mad man from the Gaderenes clearly had mental illnesses. With both of these people the mental state was associated with demon possession. As part of His earthly ministry, Jesus cast the devils out of these individuals and restored them as whole and in a right mind. However, it was not just mental illness that was associated with demonic activity but also many other diseases (blindness, deafness and dumbness). To attribute a devil behind all mental and physical illness is clearly not what happened in Jesus' time. Sometimes mental illness and other diseases were associated with demonic possession and sometimes not. Another example is seen in the second use of the word *'lunatick'* where those who were classified such were distinguished from all other illnesses including those who were *'possessed with devils'*. *"And Jesus went about all Galilee, teaching in their synagogues, and preaching the gospel of the kingdom, and healing **all manner of sickness and all manner of disease** among the people. And his fame went throughout all Syria: and they brought unto him* *that were taken with **diverse diseases and torments**, and those which were **possessed with devils**, and those which were **lunatick**, and those that had the **palsy**; and he healed them."* (Matthew 4:23-24) The Bible clearly distinguishes times when people recognised the difference between a natural mental illness and a demonic mental illness.

As a couple, we personally believe that Christians cannot be demon *possessed* but can be *oppressed* in their thinking. This is part of the spiritual battle all Christians can face at times. The Bible warns of this when the apostle Paul encourages Christians to take their stand in spiritual warfare.

> *"Finally, my brethren, be strong in the Lord, and in the power of his might. Put on the whole armour of God, that ye may be able to stand against the wiles of the devil. For we wrestle not against flesh and blood, but against principalities, against powers, against the rulers of the darkness of this world, against spiritual wickedness in high places. Wherefore take unto you the whole armour of God, that ye may be able to withstand in the evil day, and having done all, to stand."* (Ephesians 6:10-13)

The thought of being demon-possessed can plague and torment a Christian who is suffering with a mental illness. The mere thought has sent Christians on an immediate search for a deliverance ministry, only later to discover the disappointment that their bipolar was not removed.

It is wise to clearly distinguish between natural mental illness and demonic mental illness. One of the most powerful weapons God has given to us is His Word. When the scriptures are quoted in relation to the problems a demoniac is suffering, there is usually agitation and even violent reactions to the Bible. On the contrary, when the Word of God is read or quoted to those who are bipolar, generally the scriptures are a great source of help and comfort and do not cause any negative reactions.

Another phrase used in the scriptures that would also refer to the mental state of a person is *"beside himself."* This is an idiom meaning to be in such a strong emotional state that it makes you almost out of control. Both Jesus and the apostle Paul were accused of being mentally unstable due to the things they were saying. People listened to what they had to say and thought "these are the words of an insane person."

Early in the ministry of Jesus, whilst preaching and gathering a large crowd in a house, some of His friends were embarrassed and thought Jesus had 'lost it' and had gotten carried away with Himself. They thought His preaching was a sign of insanity and claimed He was *"beside himself"* and tried to take Him away. *"And when his friends heard of it, they went out to lay hold on him: for they said, **He is beside himself."** (Mark 3:21)

Under investigation by Roman officials, the apostle Paul corrected the accusation that his learning experiences had created a mental illness in his life. *"And as he thus spake for himself, Festus said with a loud voice, Paul, **thou art beside thyself; much learning doth make thee mad.** But he said, **I am not mad**, most noble Festus; but speak forth the words of truth and soberness.* " (Acts 26:24)

Almost all the references to mental illness in the Bible were perceived by others in a negative and shameful light that needed to be shunned by society. Many were often treated as outcasts from their communities. Sadly, much of this stigmatisation has been continued throughout the centuries and people with mental illness have been misunderstood, poorly treated and ostracised. It was the way people were simply classified, but thankfully they were not categorised in that light by God.

We believe a right response to people suffering with a mental illness is to pray for and encourage them, not judge them, accuse them of being 'demonised', or deny their problems. People with mental illness are not second class citizens; they are loved by God and many that we personally know have great and impressive faith in the Lord whilst struggling with very difficult problems.

I (Robert) personally think those of us who enjoy such an easy life in terms of being able to cope in our daily lives mentally without having our whole world collapse around us now and again, ought to be inspired by sufferers of bipolar and other mental illnesses. People like my wife and many others we know can be an incredible example of trusting in God, relying on His Word and grace to sustain them in a life of uncertainty no matter what state they are in each day.

However, one area that needs to be addressed is the blame shifting and non-acceptance of responsibility of sinful attitudes and actions. We all have a sinful nature which desires to sin. It is very easy for our sinful nature to cause our heart to be deceived. The heart of man does not get a good wrap in the Bible. *"The heart is deceitful above all things, and desperately wicked: who can know it?"* (Jeremiah 17:9) This is why we are admonished to protect our heart. *"Keep thy heart with all diligence; for out of it are the issues of life."* (Proverbs 4:23) The Word of God is what helps us guard our heart from being deceived. *"Thy word have I hid in mine heart, that I might not sin against thee."* (Psalm 119:11)

It is easy to gloss over sin, especially when atheistic psychologists and psychiatrists, following Freudism ideology, seek to manage their behaviours through therapy and or medication. When comparing these to their Christian counterparts using biblical principles, we need to identify what the Bible calls sin and deal with it biblically not just therapeutically as a 'mental illness'. Most of our generic mental ills are just the ills of sin, which require nothing more than repentance and faith in Christ followed by a total intent of surrendering our life over to Him and His Word, both internally and externally. We must limit mental illness to real medically understood anomalies that are different from just intense sinful cravings. We are not in any way denying that some forms of mental illness can cause a person to act in a manner for which they are inculpable, for example, in times of hallucinations and insanity.

What we are saying is we must not be too quick to diagnose sinful beliefs and behaviours as purely the result of mental illness. A person may not have any mental illness at all but may simply be reacting to the guilt and conviction which comes from breaking the laws of God. One role of the pastor and or Christian counsellor is to help a person identify if any false beliefs and sinful behaviour has them captive and then to teach them to follow the truth of God's Word. *"And the servant of the Lord must not strive; but be gentle unto all men, apt to teach, patient, In meekness instructing those that oppose themselves; if God peradventure will give them repentance to the acknowledging of the truth; And that they may recover themselves out of the snare of the devil, who are taken captive by him at his will."* (2 Timothy 2:24-26)

A Christian familiar with the New Testament, especially the Pauline epistles, notices how Paul continually speaks of the gospel indicatives then follows them up with the gospel imperatives. For example, the book of Ephesians spends the first three chapters telling us who we are in Christ and what Christ and the gospel have truly done for those in the spiritual realm. Once this is accepted, believed and received by faith by the Christian, our position in Christ is totally different. We truly are living on the victory side of life. Then we understand that *"Christ is our life"*, that we ARE seated in heavenly places IN CHRIST and that we do have access to the POWER that RAISED Jesus from the dead. Then and only then can we look to the gospel imperatives of what God can now do through us: the practical working out of our faith.

We must first understand and reckon it to be so by faith, all that God has done IN us through Christ and his death, burial and resurrection. Then we can have freedom to allow God to work THROUGH us in living a life of victory over sin and infirmities.

The book of Romans is another fine example of this approach to understanding the power available to the Christian. The first eleven chapters teach us what God has done for us and in us. Then we begin chapter 12 with great intrinsic motivation when God has Paul encourage us and challenge us to simply DO what is our reasonable service because of HIS MERCIES. *"I beseech you therefore, brethren, by the mercies of God, that ye present your bodies a living sacrifice, holy, acceptable unto God, which is your reasonable service. And be not conformed to this world: but be ye transformed by the renewing of your mind, that ye may prove what is that good, and acceptable, and perfect, will of God."* (Romans 12:1-2)

But to simply try and DO the Christian life and live the practical aspects of scripture without understanding and appropriating the power within to do these things, will lead to more and more frustration and failures for the Christian.

We don't simply focus on behaviours that need to be changed. We MUST focus and accept by faith what God has done for us in and through the cross so that we find all our significance, security, self worth and satisfaction in Jesus and our personal relationship with Him.

It is only when we do this that we can find the power to stand against the wiles of the devil and wrestle with the slanderous thoughts that have bombarded our minds making it feeble and infirmed.

Yes, medication and therapies have their place in the management of the physiological aspects of the illness. However, for freedom to be found even in the midst of mania or depressive times, knowing who you are IN Christ makes all the difference.

When considering the role of the Word of God in the life of a bipolar sufferer, there is a fundamental foundation that must be in place before dealing with bipolar disorder. First, the person has to be born again by trusting the Lord Jesus Christ as personal Saviour. Once this occurs he is then able to access the power and the understanding to deal with bipolar disorder Biblically through the work of the Holy Spirit Who lives in the believer. *"But the natural man receiveth not the things of the Spirit of God: for they are foolishness unto him: neither can he know them, because they are spiritually discerned. But he that is spiritual judgeth all things, yet he himself is judged of no man. For who hath known the mind of the Lord, that he may instruct him? But we have the mind of Christ."* (1 Corinthians 2:14-16)

After being born again, he must be willing to accept that God's Word applies to every situation in life including bipolar disorder. The scriptures are the primary means of God's communication to us to guide our lives. They provide us with wisdom to direct us in all situations. *"All scripture is given by inspiration of God, and is profitable for doctrine, for reproof, for correction, for instruction in righteousness: That the man of God may be perfect, throughly furnished unto all good works."* (2 Timothy 3:16-17) In fact one of my (Jenny) favourite verses of scripture deals with this very thought – *"Trust in the LORD with all thine heart; and lean not unto thine own understanding. In all thy ways acknowledge him, and he shall direct thy paths." (Proverbs 3:5-6)*

As a believer, I (Jenny) have learnt to try to focus on allowing Christ to control my thoughts at all times. Later in the book we will discuss the battle for the mind and the power of thought control. However, if I find myself in either a depressive mood with its sadness and hopelessness or in a manic mood feeling abnormally euphoric and full of energy, I seek to take prayerful action immediately. I cannot afford my thoughts and vain imaginations to wander into areas that would not be pleasing to God, so I seek to bring them in line with God's Word. The apostle Paul writes about the warfare of the mind and the necessity to not allow wrong thinking to gain a stronghold. *"For though we walk in the flesh, we do not war after the flesh: (For the weapons of our warfare are not carnal, but mighty through God to the pulling down of **strong holds**;) Casting down imaginations, and every high thing that exalteth itself against the knowledge of God, and bringing into captivity every thought to the obedience of Christ; And having in a readiness to revenge all disobedience, when your obedience is fulfilled." (2 Corinthians 10:3-6)*

If my thoughts are contrary to God's Word, then I must bring my thinking back in line with the Holy Spirit-produced thinking. I recall that God has given me a sound mind even though my physiological brain may be causing me bipolar moments. *"For God hath not given us the spirit of fear; but of power, and of love, and of a sound mind." (2 Timothy 1:7)*

A faithful friend of mine, Leanne Gray (*pictured right*), would sit on my bed and listen to me talk. As I would say what I was thinking (mostly negative thoughts) she would say "Don't take that thought; chuck that out of your thinking."

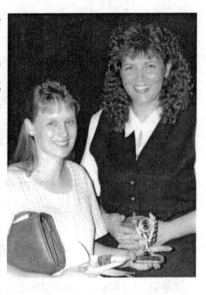

I have found it helpful to keep a diary and write down common thoughts, circumstances, seasons of the year, weather, or anything else I have found that seems to be happening when my moods swing. This becomes a good reference point for me to be ready to counter any bipolar attacks with prayer.

The Bible tells us that bipolar can't make you sin. If we sin it is because of our own sinful desires and choices. *"But every man is tempted, when he is drawn away of his own lust, and enticed. Then when lust hath conceived, it bringeth forth sin: and sin, when it is finished, bringeth forth death." (James 1:14)*

Just because I have a chemical imbalance in my brain, this is no excuse to ignore Godly counsel and/or sound advice. My brain problems cannot force me to follow my own desires and live impulsively, or move outside God-ordained sexual boundaries. It is a choice and, yes, admittedly a difficult choice when your mind and brain seem to be working against each other. I, like every other person, am commanded by God to love the Lord with ALL my heart, soul, mind and body and to love my neighbour as myself.

"And one of the scribes came, and having heard them reasoning together, and perceiving that he had answered them well, asked him, Which is the first commandment of all? And Jesus answered him, The first of all the commandments is, Hear, O Israel; The Lord our God is one Lord: **And thou shalt love the Lord thy God with all thy heart, and with all thy soul, and with all thy mind, and with all thy strength:** *this is the first commandment. And the second is like, namely this, Thou shalt love thy neighbour as thyself. There is none other commandment greater than these."* (Mark 12:28-31)

At times, when one is in a bipolar state, it can create a world of temptations. It is very easy to allow moods to control your mind and thinking. I can convince myself to trust in intuitive judgements rather than be cautious of them. The altered mood, especially in a mania state, can provide the catalyst to tempt me to throw caution to the wind and spend up big on the credit card. It became a standard joke around our home and with friends, to hide the credit card anytime I was in a manic moment. Undoubtedly, bipolar can affect my ability to make wise judgements and makes certain decisions feel so right. However, it can't make one do anything that Scripture prohibits or condemns. If I do, then it is my choice.

Although bipolar undoubtedly has a physical and medical basis, there's more to it than that. It's too easy to become fatalistic and shirk personal responsibility, saying, "It's not my fault that I have these extreme mood swings; I'm totally helpless to control them. I'm like a puppet whose strings are pulled by some invisible biochemical, bipolar puppeteer". You don't have to subscribe to the idea of being a perpetual victim of a genetic 'chemical imbalance'. My genes might predispose me to radical mood changes but that doesn't mean I'm helpless and must yield to the vulnerabilities of bipolar thinking.

I can't be filled with bitterness, grudges and unforgiveness and then use my bipolar as an excuse for these sins. I am accountable for my actions and attitudes no matter how difficult it is for me to not yield to the temptation because of my illness.

Consider a few of the ten commandments from Exodus 20:12-17 and think how foolish it is if we placed the wording *"except if you have bipolar"* after each of the commandments. Could you imagine the anarchy and damage this would cause to sufferers of bipolar and to others? This is how they would read…

> **"Honour thy father and thy mother**: that thy days may be long upon the land which the LORD thy God giveth thee, *except if you have bipolar."*

> "That shalt **not kill**, *except if you have bipolar."*

> "Thou shalt **not commit adultery**, *except if you have bipolar."*

> "Thou shalt **not steal**, *except if you have bipolar."*

> "Thou shalt **not bear false witness** against thy neighbour, *except if you have bipolar."*

> "Thou shalt **not covet** thy neighbour's house, thou shalt not covet thy neighbour's wife, nor his manservant, nor his maidservant, nor his ox, nor his ass, nor any thing that is thy neighbour's, *except if you have bipolar."*

We cannot use bipolar disorder as an excuse to sin. When God gives a command or a prohibition in His Word it speaks to everyone who hears. If those with bipolar disorder were exempt, we would all be exempt because none of us has a perfectly functioning brain. We are all human beings who live before a perfect God in imperfect bodies.

What we need to access is the grace of God to help in times of need and temptation. We all need God's grace to live as His children and we can all receive that grace when we come to Him and ask. Grace is that ability that God gives believers to do what they normally and naturally couldn't do or to not do what they normally would. As believers we have access to God's throne through prayer to ask for grace to help us in our struggles and temptations. Jesus knows what it is like to be tempted. *"Seeing then that we have a great high priest, that is passed into the heavens, Jesus the Son of God, let us hold fast our profession. For we have not an high priest which cannot be touched with the feeling of our infirmities; but was in all points tempted like as we are, yet without sin. Let us therefore come boldly unto the throne of grace, that we may obtain mercy, and find grace to help in time of need." (Hebrews 4:14-16)*

The apostle Paul spoke of God's grace enabling him to live with his physical infirmity. *"And lest I should be exalted above measure through the abundance of the revelations, there was given to me a thorn in the flesh, the messenger of Satan to buffet me, lest I should be exalted above measure. For this thing I besought the Lord thrice, that it might depart from me. And he said unto me, **My grace is sufficient for thee**: for my strength is made perfect in weakness. Most gladly therefore will I rather glory in my infirmities, that the power of Christ may rest upon me. Therefore I take pleasure in infirmities, in reproaches, in necessities, in persecutions, in distresses for Christ's sake: for when I am weak, then am I strong." (2 Corinthians 12:7-10)*

As Christians, we believe the Bible portrays us as both physical and spiritual. However, psychiatric theories tend to see human beings as merely physical and do not consider the spiritual realm. The scriptures clearly teach us that we are all responsible for our moral decisions. Brain problems cannot erase this accountability. *"For we* must **all** appear before the judgment seat of Christ; that **every one** may receive the things done in his body, according to that he hath done, **whether it be good or bad.**" (2 Corinthians 5:10)

What bipolar disorder does is cause one's mind to race, be unable to sleep yet be energetic and at times, makes your thoughts chaotic. But notice that these are not explicitly moral problems. They are neither commanded nor condemned in scripture. They can, as I suggested earlier, create the opportunity for a plethora of temptations; but the brain problems themselves cannot make us sin. We make choices.

If we know we have sinned against God, the treatment for sin is confession. Start by confessing your sins to God. The Bible tells us, "*If we confess our sins, he is faithful and just to forgive us our sins, and to cleanse us from all unrighteousness.*" (1 John 1:9) Dare to believe that because of Jesus' death and resurrection we can actually be forgiven for every wrong we have done.

Whether we suffer from bipolar or not, Christians must all strive to be conformed to the image of His Son, to walk as He walked and let the mind of Christ be in us.

> "*For whom he did foreknow, he also did predestinate to **be conformed to the image** of his Son, that he might be the firstborn among many brethren.*" (Romans 8:29)

> "*He that saith he abideth in him ought himself also so to **walk, even as he walked**.*" (1 John 2:6)

> "*Let this **mind be in you**, which was also in Christ Jesus:*" (Philippians 2:5)

Because bipolar messes with brain chemicals and thinking processes, it is vital that we make a conscious effort to guard our thoughts. We must increase our prayer life asking God to guide us and seek counsel to validate decisions that we are contemplating. One good prayer to pray is written in the Psalms. *"Search me, O God, and know my heart: try me, and know my thoughts: And see if there be any wicked way in me, and lead me in the way everlasting." (Psalm 139:23-24)*

No matter what temptation may come our way, whether we have bipolar or not, God has promised to always make a *"way to escape"* the temptation. We just have to choose to take the escape route. *"There hath no temptation taken you but such as is common to man: but God is faithful, who will not suffer you to be tempted above that ye are able; but will with the temptation also make a **way to escape**, that ye may be able to bear it." (1 Corinthians 10:13)*

Nothing can keep us from living the life the Lord desires of us. Even in moments of bipolar we can find a *"way to escape"*. For me (Jenny) the main temptations to sin in my life have been internal issues more than external ones. It seems to be attitudes and negative thoughts that plague me especially in my depressive lows.

God has made several escape routes available for me that kept me from yielding to the temptation of wallowing in self-pity or getting angry at others for their seeming lack of understanding.

Some of these ways of escape have been:

- **Scriptures**

  I use a daily devotional called "Daily Light"[13] which is simply a compilation of scriptures for each day. Various verses dealing with fear and trusting in God have become a source of comfort during instability. They provide me the anchor

---

13 An online copy of this devotional can be found - http://www.dailylightdevotional.org/

for my soul and right my thinking like the ballast on a ship. The spiritual problems exposed especially through the mania episodes, such as impulsiveness, unwillingness to seek or hear counsel or the tendency to go down a path that has painful consequences are addressed in the wisdom literature of scripture. I have found the wisdom principles and precepts in the book of Proverbs in the Old Testament and James in the New Testament have been a wonderful source of stability as I follow Biblical advice.

- *Spouse*

To have an understanding spouse is an incredible blessing in moments of bipolar. Robert has his moments of frustration with me, but his ability to notice my mania mood swings when I don't - whilst I don't like to hear it - has been helpful to get medical treatment earlier. In addition to this he provides me with a sounding board for my ideas and advises me on courses of actions to take, even if this means to rest when I feel like racing.

- *Singing*

I recall a time when I was very sick and a shadow of darkness had overwhelmed me. I was ready to give up and saw no hope of recovery. I had withdrawn all affection from Robert and my family and would just continually cry. Robert sat on the end of our bed and picked up his guitar and started to play and sing to me. He sang a song written by Dottie Rambo called, "Too much to gain to lose". The lyrics and heartfelt words of my husband were a great escape to me that day and gave me a glimmer of hope.

Too many miles behind me
Too many trials are through
Too many tears help me to remember
There's too much to gain to lose
Too many sunsets lie behind the mountain
Too many rivers my feet have walked through
Too many treasures are waiting over yonder
There's too much to gain to lose.[14]

- **Selflessness**

Do you ever hold 'pity parties' for yourself that go for an extended period of time? Do your family and friends walk on proverbial 'egg shells' when they are around you during one of your moods? Do you ever harbour grudges and become angry and unforgiving to others who seem to not care or understand? I have answered "Yes" to each of these questions and recognised that I became consumed with myself and my illness. I needed to humbly look to God and die to self. Humility is a glowing exit sign in the emotional darkness that provides an escape route to selfishness and self centeredness.

- **Sovereignty**

Christians believe that God is always in control and makes no mistakes. His ways are perfect and His counsels are unshakeable. While God cannot control our free wills, He does have purposes and plans for our lives. God can use circumstances and situations to get our attention and change our focus and attitudes. Many times we believe God has used people and circumstantial events to provide divine escapes

14 "Too Much To Gain To Lose" by Dottie Rambo can be seen online https://www.youtube.com/watch?v=rzlvjavDPMI

from potentially damaging and destructive times. Throughout my sickness, I have received phone calls or personal visits from people just in the moment of time when I was ready to give up. During a difficult time of deciding whether or not I should undergo electric shock treatment, Robert came across a book called, "Broken Minds"[15] written by a pastor who himself had undergone the treatment. The book helped answer so many questions and gave us a peace from God we hadn't had before. Many of these small signs of God's hand on our lives have helped us trust in His sovereign power more and more. We have found if we continually fear the Lord and depend on Him for guidance, we find the wisdom we need, at either pole, that have helped us avoid potential disasters in our marriage and ministry lives. In light of the mood swings and cycles I desperately needed wisdom and knowledge from God to provide a balance in my thinking. *"The fear of the LORD is the beginning of wisdom: and the knowledge of the holy is understanding." (Proverbs 9:10)*

- **Submission**

Hearing advice is one thing; taking the advice is another. When a doctor tells you what you don't want to hear but you submit to it anyway, it is an escape route from what may have been another crash. When a loving trusted friend throws cold water on your 'fire' of wonderful creativity and quenches the manic urge, that's a great escape. This is why my trusted counsellors in life have become an invaluable source of help and direction. The Bible again reminds us of the need to seek counsel. Think of a counsellor as a coach who reinforces good habits and practices and seeks to remove bad ones.

15 *Broken Minds*, Steve & Robyn Bloem, Kregal Publications, Grand Rapids, Michigan, USA 2005

*"Where no **counsel** is, the people fall: but in the multitude of **counsellors** there is safety."* *(Proverbs 11:14)*

*"The way of a fool is right in his own eyes: but he that hearkeneth unto **counsel** is wise."* *(Proverbs 12:15)*

*"Without counsel purposes are disappointed: but in the multitude of **counsellors** they are established."* *(Proverbs 15:22)*

*"Hear **counsel**, and receive instruction, that thou mayest be wise in thy latter end. There are many devices in a man's heart; nevertheless the **counsel** of the LORD, that shall stand."* *(Proverbs 19:20-21)*

Do you know two or three wise people who will give you honest and helpful counsel? Ensure you have people who you can talk with and get in the habit of following your advisor's counsel whenever at least two agree: *"...In the mouth of two or three witnesses shall every word be established."* *(2 Corinthians 13:1)* This will become a profound protection for you in your life at either polar end.

- **Strategies**

Pre-planning as much as you can provides escape routes during the foggy days. For example, simply planning your meals for a week helps take away additional stress and anxiety when you hit a low. I have a shopping list for three weeks of meals that I refer to when I simply can't think straight. Having this strategy in my weaker moments has been a great escape.

- *Sleep*

  Elijah needed sleep during his times of depression and afterward was able to deal with the issues at hand. Sometimes the greatest escape is to get proper bed rest and allow your body and brain to recuperate.

- *Sequesters*

  Time out, whether in hospital or away with family and friends has provided much needed escapes to allow time for me to manage my bipolar. In January 2016 I spent two glorious weeks in Tasmania with my twin sister Maree and the change of scenery and time away from regular duties was therapeutic.

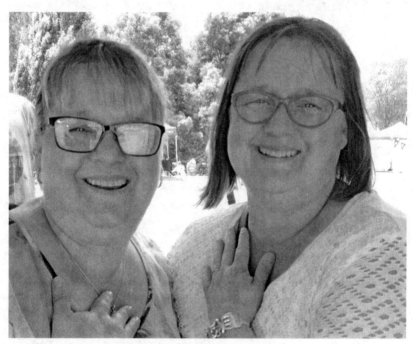

Jenny and her twin sister Maree.

CHAPTER 7

IS IT WRONG TO TAKE MEDICINE?

DRUGS

A question we are often asked is whether it is right or wrong for a Christian to take medication for bipolar.

The use of psychiatric medications is a topic of controversy that is not unique to Christian circles. Many people have legitimate questions and concerns about the effectiveness of the drugs. A cursory search of the internet will reveal several academics, naturopaths and medical professionals writing critiques of the use of psychoactive medications.

Generally, people who experience any form of bipolar will consult with a psychiatrist or qualified physician and will be prescribed some psychiatric medication. There are many new medications that appear regularly and I (Jenny) have been exposed to many of them since 1993. Most of them are a form of Lithium or medications that have also been used to control seizures.

The nagging question that plagues many Christians is whether they should try medication or not. Some feel that to take medication is a sign of weakness and lack of faith in God, while others see it as a blessing from God. Who is right?

In one study conducted in the United States of America, nearly half of evangelical, fundamentalist, or born-again Christians, believe prayer and Bible study alone can overcome serious mental illness. [16] The prevailing thought is that we are, as a society, overmedicated and that carries an even greater stigma for those inside the church.

For us as a couple, we decided to look to the scriptures and consider if God would endorse the use of medicines or whether taking them was an indication of a lack of faith and therefore displeasing to the Lord. Obviously, the Bible does not mention the use of synthetic drugs specifically, as they are a result of the constant advancement in new research and modern technology. However, many Bible authors do refer to the use of other natural substances as medicinal treatments to aid in the healing and recovery process.

In one instance in the Old Testament, the then king of Judah, Hezekiah, was sick and close to death. The prophet Isaiah was instructed by God to prescribe the king a form of medicinal treatment which healed him of his sickness. *"In those days was Hezekiah **sick unto death**. And the prophet Isaiah the son of Amoz came to him, and said unto him, Thus saith the LORD, Set thine house in order; for thou shalt die, and not live. Then he turned his face to the wall, and prayed unto the LORD, saying, I beseech thee, O LORD, remember now how I have walked before thee in truth and with a perfect heart, and have done that which is good in thy sight. And Hezekiah wept sore. And it came to pass, afore Isaiah was gone out into the middle court, that the word of the LORD came to him, saying, Turn again, and tell Hezekiah the captain of my people, Thus saith the LORD, the God of David thy father, I have heard thy prayer, I have seen thy tears: behold, **I will heal thee**: on the third day thou shalt go up unto the house of the LORD. And I will add unto thy days fifteen years; and I will deliver thee and*

---

16 http://www.christianitytoday.com/edstetzer/2014/june/mental-illness-and-christian.html

this city out of the hand of the king of Assyria; and I will defend this city for mine own sake, and for my servant David's sake. And Isaiah said, **Take a lump of figs. And they took and laid it on the boil, and he recovered.**" (2 Kings 20:1-7)

In endorsing the use of medicine, King Solomon compares a happy heart to the use of medicine that does good to the recipient. "*A merry heart doeth good like a medicine: but a broken spirit drieth the bones.*" (Proverbs 17:22)

The prophet Jeremiah, in speaking of the judgement of God upon the nation of Israel, uses a metaphor which confirms the practice of healing medicines. "*For thus saith the LORD, Thy bruise is incurable, and thy wound is grievous. There is none to plead thy cause, that thou mayest be bound up: thou hast no healing medicines.*" (Jeremiah 30:12-13)

Again, Jeremiah metaphorically makes reference to healing through medicine and questions why the physician and medicines were not being used to help in recovery. "*Is there no balm in Gilead; is there no physician there? why then is not the health of the daughter of my people recovered?*" (Jeremiah 8:22)

The apostle Paul prescribed a medical remedy for a young man with a persistent stomach complaint. "*Drink no longer water, but use a little wine for thy stomach's sake and thine often infirmities.*" (1 Timothy 5:23)

Whilst travelling in many of his missionary journeys, the apostle Paul had a doctor as his travelling companion. Luke, was affectionately referred to by Paul as "*the beloved physician*" (Colossians 4:14). Even in his last days on the earth, when many had abandoned him, Paul said *"Only Luke is with me."* *(2 Timothy 4:11)* No doubt Doctor Luke helped him in his physical ailments until the end.

The most convincing thought for us that God endorses the use of medicines to aid in healing are the words of our Saviour the Lord Jesus Christ. *"When Jesus heard it, he saith unto them, They that are whole have no need of the physician, but they that are sick: I came not to call the righteous, but sinners to repentance."* *(Mark 2:17)*

From these scriptures and prayer, coupled with counsel from trusted pastors and medical professionals, we believe that medication was one of the blessings God provided to aid with or maintain my well-being whilst living with bipolar disorder. I (Jenny) am really conscious to allow Robert and others around me who know me well to bring it to my attention if I am becoming 'unhealthy' in my moods. They can often notice signs of a bipolar episode earlier than I can and see changes in my behaviour and countenance before I even notice. At times, an adjustment in my medication will help me stay balanced and stop an episode occurring.

Before having been diagnosed with bipolar disorder I needed very little medication in life. Maybe a paracetamol tablet once or twice a year. I exercised regularly, ate healthy food and managed and organised the home. I taught Sunday school at church, helped Robert run the Youth Group on Friday evening and assisted in our Christian school. I lived a full and happy life. Once bipolar became a part of my life, medication helped me maintain a balance in my moods and enabled me to have a semblance of my 'normal' life that I was used to.

I have always strived to keep a daily diary of my mood, medications/ amounts and any triggers that may have started an episode. This has been a great help to my doctor and psychiatrist during times of consultation to assess the effectiveness of my treatment.

As a couple, we do, indeed, believe that medication is called for at times. Having said that, we also believe there is a distinction between a spiritual struggle and a mental illness that we must keep in mind. In our experience we have encountered a few people who were readily prescribed psychiatric medications for issues that appeared to us to be matters of the heart, soul and mind, not a chemical imbalance in the brain. We think the major reason why people jump solely to chemical solutions is usually because they don't understand how to treat the problem any other way. In chapter 15 we discuss the differences between the various types of depression including the possible causes and treatments for each.

If a person has a mental illness, which is a physiological reality, then we definitely believe they need to seek medicinal treatment. However, if a person is struggling with a fear, bitterness, a sin, grief or any other host of issues, having people who can provide Godly counsel and encouragement from God's Word may be all the medicine that person needs to help them through a depressive moment.

There should be no shame in a person being diagnosed with bipolar and needing to take medication to aid in their well-being. We wouldn't shame someone for getting diabetes or high blood pressure. Why do we shame someone for having a chemical imbalance that leads him or her to a lifelong struggle with bipolar?

We totally believe what the apostle Paul wrote to the Philippians, *"I can do all things through Christ which strengtheneth me." (Philippians 4:13)* But that doesn't mean that we don't need the support of family, friends and medical help to do those things. God can use *"all things"* to help us do *"all things."*

We both believe that God is able to miraculously heal a person of their mental illness, if He chooses to do so. Some may go from doctor to doctor and spend a fortune seeking help only to find none, then God steps in and performs a miracle. There is an event in the life of Jesus where this happened:

> "And a certain woman, which had an issue of blood twelve years, And had suffered many things of many physicians, and had spent all that she had, and was nothing bettered, but rather grew worse, When she had heard of Jesus, came in the press behind, and touched his garment. For she said, If I may touch but his clothes, I shall be whole. And straightway the fountain of her blood was dried up; and she felt in her body that she was healed of that plague." (Mark 5:25-29)

While not for everyone, I (Jenny) probably wouldn't be alive if it weren't for the medications I take. I have always maintained that medication allows me to function at a more balanced level and I suspect it has saved my life more than once. It was God who led me to the right people to help me with the correct medication.

One of the most helpful things family members can do for a person suffering from a bipolar disorder is to help them keep taking their medication. For me, Robert has been a great support and encouragement in this regard. I also have my Pharmacist prepare a "Webster pack" which allows me to keep track of the day and time I need to take my meds. This has been very helpful, especially in the down times when my memory is not good and my thoughts are foggy. Ensure you always check your pack for accuracy of the prescribed medications.

Bipolar disorder is difficult to deal with, yet it is also true that this problem can usually be effectively managed with proper professional care over the long term. Medication, psychotherapy (for me this includes spiritual counsel) and lifestyle changes minimise and overcome the most devastating effects of this disorder and enable the sufferer to generally live a normal life at home, work, school and church. However, the treatment must be planned for the rest of the sufferer's life and it nearly always involves taking medication for many years. It took me several years to finally accept this as part of my personal journey.

The current drug treatments for bipolar disorder typically include what are referred to as mood stabilizers—usually lithium carbonate. Some, but not all, anticonvulsants may be combined with lithium or with other anticonvulsants for optimal effect. Some commonly used anticonvulsants include carbamazepine (Tegretol), lamotrigine (Lamictal) and valproic acid (Depakote). Depending on a number of factors such as the specifics of the person's symptoms and the stage of the disorder, the doctors may also prescribe antipsychotic, antidepressant, or anti-anxiety medication. While medications do not work perfectly, they help a substantial percentage of people. Approximately 50 to 70 percent of people in a manic state are helped by lithium.[17] Whilst Lithium is an effective mood stabilizing medication, it can change your thyroid functions. Bipolar patients may be at more risk of thyroid abnormalities and it is essential your doctor monitors your lithium levels through regular blood tests to ensure you remain in a therapeutic range.

Strangely, during my final two pregnancies I was not able to take any bipolar medication and thankfully was episode-free throughout the entire nine months each time. Apparently the rapid change in hormones in my body enabled me to have no signs of bipolar. At first, after the birth of my fourth child, Timothy, I thought I no longer had bipolar and would never have to take medication again. However,

---

17 http://lifecounsel.org/pub_hall_understandingBipolar.html

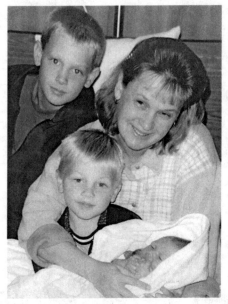

within a month or so, the bipolar cycle returned with a mania episode followed by the all-familiar 'crash'. Exactly the same circumstances happened with my last pregnancy with Jonathan. Sadly, because I went back on to medication I was unable to breastfeed my last two babies. One doctor cheekily suggested I stay pregnant all the time!

Whilst medication is a wonderful thing it is not without its shortcomings. I have been on a large number of medications for bipolar for the most part of twenty years. There have been times when I have sought to wean myself off medication. Sometimes, during hypermania moments while enjoying being on a 'high', I have taken my pills grudgingly even considering ceasing to take medication all together. Then during the dark moments of depression there have been times I desperately gulped them down as if my life literally depended on them. My advice is to talk to your support people about any consideration of ceasing to take medication. When someone comes off these medications it can have a very serious effect on the body. A person's life can be threatened. These kinds of medical decisions, where the health and safety of a human being are at stake, must be left to medical professionals.

There was another occasion, besides during my pregnancies, where I went almost a year without an episode. Being a person who was rather opposed to taking medication, I convinced my doctor that I was ready to gradually come off my meds and to my elation he agreed for me to get off my medication. Yes! It took me a year to gradually reduce the amounts of each tablet, as going off some medications 'cold turkey' is not a good strategy at all and can create other health problems: relapse, major side effects, enhanced suicidal tendencies or even death!

Finally in August of 2009 I was medication free and two months passed with no episodes. In October, Robert and I went on an amazing week's trip to Perth, Western Australia for a Bible Conference. It was toward the end of the week when I started to vomit. At first we thought it was food poisoning. Then with the vomiting came the crying for no apparent reason. We returned back home to Rockhampton and I was still feeling sick in the stomach. Over the course of a month I had lost 15kg and still had pain in the intestines. My doctor organised for tests to be carried out to determine if there was a problem in my stomach or intestines. The results came back negative. In some way I had hoped there was a positive result that would explain my discomfort.

Whilst in hospital in November for continual stomach pain it was suggested that the cause may be because of coming off medication and hopefully it would all settle down. I came out of the ten day stint in hospital and did okay for a while. Then just before Christmas I was back in hospital with intestine pain again. More tests were ordered and still the results came back clear. It was at this point the doctors consulted with my psychiatrist and concluded my bipolar was back and affected the second largest nervous system in our bodies – my stomach. This news hit me like a tonne of bricks and floored me. I rang Robert to tell him to hurry to the hospital. When Robert arrived and entered my hospital room I told him, amidst my crying and sobbing, that my bipolar was back. Within a few weeks of taking medication again my stomach and intestine issues disappeared. Sadly, I developed restless legs and had weight gain as a side effect. The medication had slowed my metabolism down and I was not burning off the calories like I was before. In 2013 I was diagnosed with type II diabetes which then added an additional burden to my life – daily sugar level testing.

During times when I have been in hospital I've been on many cocktails of medicines and the physical side-effects have been terrible: tremors so bad that I couldn't hold cutlery or brush my hair, a constant twitching of my tongue, vomiting, inability to walk in a straight line, blurred vision, weight gain, memory and concentration problems, constantly drenched in sweat, vivid nightmares, excessive sedation and having a mouth as dry as a desert so my throat was constantly sore.

I'm glad to say that when my mood sufficiently improves after severe episodes the doses and combinations are tweaked and the side effects settle.

These side effects may seem terrible, but I have weighed the pros and cons and the quality of life for me is better on medication than off. I have come to accept when I am a little run down that I have to go slower in undertaking tasks, but I can still get them done. If I'm sewing, beading, knitting, card-making or scrapbooking I just take my time and work with the tremors in my hand.

I take medication as one of the treatments for my bipolar; however, I recognise that brain medicine is not an exact science. Whilst medication might help contain my moods; growth in godliness certainly will. As I have grown in my understanding of God and in my spiritual life, Godly wisdom has helped limit the damage done during a bipolar episode. Nonetheless, there is no sure way to erase the possibility of future occurrences but I can try to minimise the negative consequences.

Even though I have a serious chronic medical condition, I can be an active agent in maintaining my mental well-being. I readily acknowledge that medication is a non-negotiable necessity for me. However, I also know that attitude makes a crucial difference in my mental and emotional well-being. Indeed, meds are absolutely necessary and make up probably 50 percent of what helps me overcome the mood war. The other 50 percent of the battle taking place 'between my ears' requires developing stress and life-management skills and cultivating my inner life with God. I have discovered that attitude has a lot to do with maintaining my mental well-being. Motivational speaker, Zig Ziglar once said, "It's not your aptitude but rather your attitude that determines your altitude."

Should you try medication for bipolar disorder? Obviously you need to consult with your medical professionals but I have found that generally you have nothing to lose and something to gain. At worst, you will have unwanted side effects or the medication will be ineffective. At best, you will be less prone to the mood cycles or the more intense highs. Bipolar has many symptoms and affects people differently and what is required for each person will differ according to individual needs. Make this a serious matter of prayer and ask the Lord to give you peace in your decision. *"And let the peace of God rule in your hearts, to the which also ye are called in one body; and be ye thankful."* (Colossians 3:15)

In my experience, I can either choose not to take medication and be constantly unwell, probably spending a lot of time in hospital and not functioning much at all or I can choose to live the best I can with this illness, which includes taking medication. For now I choose the second option.

CHAPTER 8

SHOCK TREATMENT

DARKNESS

Electroconvulsive therapy or ECT is a procedure performed under the direct supervision of a psychiatrist to treat certain psychiatric conditions. It involves passing a carefully controlled electrical current through the brain which induces a seizure. The treatment affects the brain's activity and aims to relieve severe depressive and psychotic symptoms. At the time of writing this book, I (Jenny) have had three bouts of ECT.

The initial clinical trial of ECT was performed by Ugo Cerletti and Lucino Bini at the University of Rome in 1938. The therapeutic use of electricity was not unique to ECT. There is evidence that Ancient Romans used the current generated by electric eels for the treatment of headaches, gout and to assist in obstetrical procedures. I am glad they don't use electric eels today!

The recent history of the therapeutic use of electricity dates to 1744 when the journal entitled "Electricity and Medicine" was first published. It was claimed here that electric stimuli could be curative for "neurologic and mental cases of paralysis and epilepsy" J.B. LeRoy in the 1755 edition of "Electricity and Medicine" detailed a case of hysterical blindness which was cured with three applications of electric shock. In 1752, Benjamin Franklin recorded the use of an "electro static machine to cure a woman of hysterical fits." By the mid 19th century the use of electrotherapy had so progressed that G.B.C. Duchenne (often referred to as the Father of Electrotherapy) would say, "No sincere neurologist could practice without the use of electrotherapy."[18]

We had only ever heard of and seen the media reports and movies depicting all types of horror stories connected to the use of shock treatment in Mental Health Institutions. One such movie was Ken Kesey's "One Flew over the Cuckoo's Nest" in which patients were shown as being given ECT without general anaesthetic or muscle relaxant (a procedure which can lead to vertebral fractures). So, when it was first suggested to Robert and me as a treatment to consider, we were both very sceptical. We have since found out that modern day ECT is safe and effective. For most people undergoing the procedure

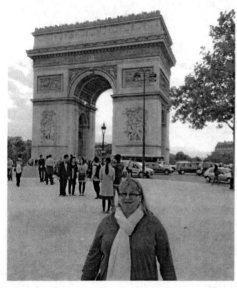

it has proved to relieve symptoms of the most severe forms of depression more effectively than medication or therapy. The only downside to ECT is that because it is an intrusive procedure it can cause some memory problems and should be used only when absolutely necessary. There are sections of life now of which I have no recollection, which saddens

At the Arc of Triumph, Paris   me at times. Robert will talk

18 For more information see "An historical review of electroconvulsive therapy" by Dr. Bruce Wright – www.jdc.jefferson.edu/cgi

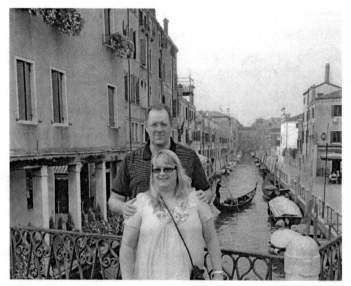

Venice, Italy

about an event in our past - a holiday though Europe that we took together in 2013 - and as much as I try to remember, I have little or no memory of sections of it.

It was after another severe low episode that my then psychiatrist suggested I get a second opinion on my condition and possibly have ECT. The closest hospital at the time that would perform the procedure was in Brisbane about eight hours away. On the 4th March, 2011, Robert and I travelled to Brisbane and I was admitted to the New Farm Mental Health Hospital for assessment and possible ECT treatment.

During my 19 day stay in hospital, the consulting psychiatrist placed me on two new medications Zaldox and Pristiq. Within a week I had bounced back to a state of normality. While we were there in New Farm, ECT was thoroughly explained to us both. It is thought that ECT works by increasing the amount of certain neurotransmitters which have a mood regulatory and antipsychotic effect. The exact mechanism is not fully known. No one knows for sure why it is effective in treating some forms of mental illness but it is thought the procedure is like a "reset button" for the brain. It is reported to have an 80 percent success rate with patients.

I returned home on the 22nd March and was functioning well but began to develop a severe twitching in my tongue and face tremors as a side effect to the new medication. By early April my bipolar struck again and I was bed-ridden and back to where I was before, maybe even a little worse.

It was then we had to seriously consider whether ECT would be an option. It was at this time that Robert was reading the book "*Broken Minds*" that I referred to in the previous chapter. The book was an incredible blessing and source of reassurance to us both as it detailed Steve's journey with mental illness and how ECT helped him.

> "*Twice I have undergone a program of between nine and twelve treatments. Both times I began improving after one treatment, and both times I was feeling noticeably better after three. It is well worth considering if a doctor suggests it as a treatment possibility. I will gladly choose this option if my depression rises to the level where suicidal thoughts and plans are present. The first time I tried E.C.T., my depression had been horrible. Excruciating pain literally brought me to my knees in the office of the medical doctor to whom I had been referred. When he highly recommended the treatments, I readily accepted.*"[19]

19 *Broken Minds*, Steve & Robyn Bloem, Kregal Publications, Grand Rapids, Michigan, USA 2005 Page 130

Robert sought counsel from a dear friend and mentor, Pastor Doug Fisher who helped in processing all the information and gave us some much needed spiritual guidance.

After much prayer and pondering of all we had read and been advised of, we decided to go ahead with ECT. For the next 26 days from the 8th April to the 3rd May I was admitted back into New Farm Mental Health Hospital for treatment. The plan was to complete twelve treatments of ECT over a four week period.

The day of my first procedure I removed all my jewellery and was told to remove my nail polish as it could interfere with some monitoring devices. I had washed my hair the night before and wore some loose fitting clothes. I was wheeled down to an operating theatre by the nursing staff and awaited my first shock treatment. I was nervous yet trusting in the Lord that He was watching over me. My biggest fear was losing my memory and waking up not knowing who I was or where I was.

I was then given an injection of two drugs, an anaesthetic and a muscle relaxant, to reduce the risk of body spasms and hypoxia (oxygen deficiency). Whilst I was anaesthetised a small electrical current was passed between two electrodes placed on my head for about three seconds inducing a generalised tonic-clonic seizure for up to one minute. Electrodes are either attached to both sides of the head (bilateral) or to just one side (unilateral), usually the non-dominant, in order to reduce the risk of cognitive side-effects. The whole procedure through to recovery lasted about 30 minutes. I was taken back to my room and fell asleep for several hours.

When I awoke Robert was there waiting for me. My hair was a mess as thick gel had been used on the area where the electrode paddles were placed. My jaw was sore and I had muscular pain throughout my body. Then came the vomiting. Every time I had a treatment I had severe vomiting following, as a reaction to the anaesthetic. During the whole process Robert kept a daily journal and recorded everything we talked about before the treatment. After the treatment we'd go over the diary, but I'd have no recollection of any of the previous day's diary entries. I was only able to physically handle eight treatments and then I decided to go home. I felt well enough to leave and just wanted to get back home.

Unfortunately, ECT is not a permanent fix, nor does it stand alone. From my experience and from conversations with friends and other patients, nearly all who have the treatment eventually relapse, often within six months. It is important to follow up with medications or occasional 'maintenance' treatments of ECT.

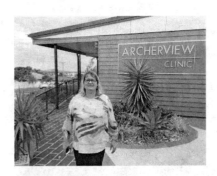
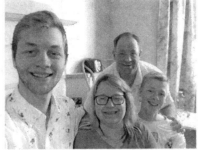
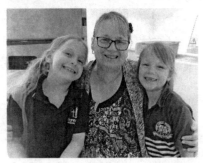
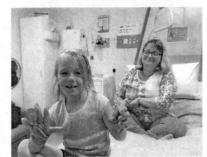

Enjoying the visits

For me I didn't opt for another round of ECT until November 2014 due to the side effects from the first time. However, with improvements in the program and under the supervision of a new psychiatrist I have undergone two more treatments of ECT since my stay in New Farm. Thankfully a new Mental Health hospital was opened in the city where I live and I was able to have the procedure there. This allowed all my children and family to be able to come visit me whilst I was an inpatient.

I (Robert) believe I have seen some improvement in Jenny's condition every time she has had ECT. Without question there have been some memory loss issues, nausea and vomiting. However, the treatment did seem to break the cycle of bipolar each time and pulled her out of her depression at the time. The second ECT required only seven of the twelve treatments before Jenny responded and bounced back. The third time Jenny had ten of the twelve treatments.

The most frustrating side effect for me is my memory loss as I (Jenny) mentioned before. My children affectionately call me 'Dory', from off the movie "Finding Nemo", because of my short term memory loss. In 2013, Robert and I travelled to Spain, England, Germany, Italy and Singapore. Just recently he showed me a photograph of himself and a hundred-year-old Spanish man standing together in the famous Plaza Mayor (Main Plaza) in Salamanca, Spain. I have no memory of being there or of taking the photo. Our son Joshua reminded me of his first part-time job when he was pushing trolleys[20] at a local supermarket. He was due to finish work at 8.00 p.m. and I had forgotten to pick him up from work and left him stranded for a couple of hours. As we laughed together about this I had to tell him I have no memory of the neglectful parenting event.

20 Trolleys are Shopping carts for all our American friends!

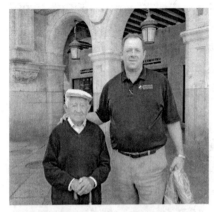

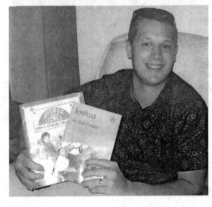

Top: Robert with the hundred-year-old Spanish man in Salamanca, Spain

Below: Joshua holding books from his childhood

In recent years modern science has come up with an alternative to ECT. It is a non-invasive procedure called repetitive Transcranial Magnetic Stimulation (TMS), but it by no means is a sure, effective treatment in depression. It involves the application of a magnetic stimulus to the brain and the effect on neurones is similar to that of ECT (depolarising) but without causing a seizure. Treatment can be undertaken without having to be anaesthetised or have a muscle relaxant. It can be done as an outpatient and the main side effect is only a mild headache. I (Jenny) have not personally had this method of treatment and have only spoken to friends who have been undergoing treatment. They have reported the treatment to be effective for them.

CHAPTER 9

LIVING WITH A PERSON WITH BIPOLAR

DISILLUSIONMENT

In 2009 Jenny was in Brisbane at New Farm Mental Health hospital for a period of two months. I (Robert) would fly down to Brisbane every week and spend time with her and then return home on the weekends to take care of our three children who were living at home at the time (Joshua, Timothy and Jonathan). I would then preach on the Sunday for our church congregation at Lighthouse Baptist Church and return to Brisbane first thing Monday morning after the boys got off to school.

It was during one of my weekend times back at home that our youngest child, JJ (Jonathan), who was eight at the time, came into my bedroom crying. He snuggled up beside me as we sat on the bed, laid his head on my chest and sniffled "When is Mum coming home?" His little heart just wanted his mummy back: the one who held him, who read to him book after book after book. He wanted the mother who played games with him and helped him with his homework. He wanted the security of his mum who stayed by his side until he fell asleep, who said, "I love you" and kissed him on the cheek. He longed for his mum who made his lunches the way only a mother can, who was the comforting face after a tough day at school. He wanted his

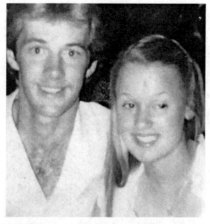

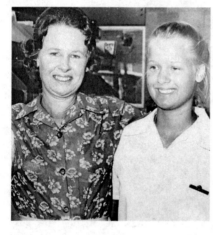

Top: High-school sweethearts!

Below: Jenny and her mother, Barbara

mummy and there was nothing I could do for him except cry with him and try to reassure him mummy would be home soon.

As a husband who has lived with a wife who has had bipolar for such a long time, I have had my own share of struggles that I have had to wrestle with. There were the many frustrations of trying to work out what was wrong with my wife to the feeling of absolute helplessness and inadequacy as I kissed her goodbye when leaving her hospital bedside.

Jenny and I met as high-school sweethearts and thoroughly enjoyed our time together all through High School and into our early young adult years. We were married in 1984 and settled on the Sunshine Coast in Queensland, where I was working in a law office at the time. We were able to build our first home on the Sunshine Coast and as a young couple with our first child (Ben) and my legal career developing, we couldn't have been happier.

In 1987 we relocated to a little country town where I attended a night Bible Institute for a few years. I began working in a legal office in Ipswich and later transferred to work in local Government offices. God blessed us with two more children, our daughter Anna and our next son Joshua. Our time in the country region was a total change of pace and environment from living on the Sunshine Coast. Jenny and I settled into country living, with our chooks (chickens) and the neighbour's cattle lowing next door. We were a happy contented little family looking forward to the prospect of eventually serving the Lord full-time in ministry somewhere.

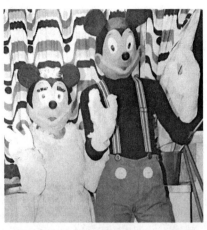

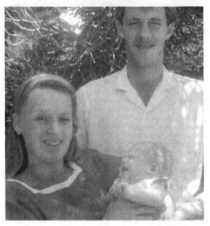

Top: Jenny made the costumes in high-school

Below: New parents

As already mentioned in chapter one, that 'somewhere' came in the form of Youth Pastor in Rockhampton in 1993. We again relocated, this time to a regional country city. The Lord provided work at the then Rockhampton City Council, which gave me a great opportunity to learn about the inner workings of the city and meet key people within the community. It was work in the day and ministry and family in the evenings and weekends.

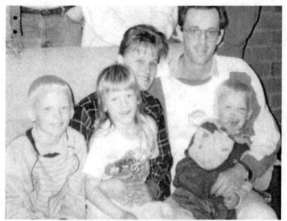

At this point in time, Jenny and I had decided to home school Ben and Anna who were 7 and 5 years old respectively. Everything seemed to be going well for us and our marriage and family life was hassle-free. We were both actively involved co-ordinating a Friday night youth program at church and volunteering in various roles in the Sunday church ministries.

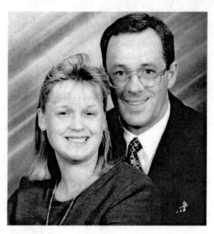

Top: Ben, Anna, Jenny, Robert and Joshua in 1992

Below: Jenny and Robert in 1999

It was within the year in 1993 that things began to change. As we mentioned earlier in the book, bipolar entered our lives. Had the disorder been lying dormant and suddenly become active? Jenny had a wonderful family home with no indication of mental illness throughout her childhood and teenage years. Her life was filled with many sports, with gymnastics and surfing being her favourite. From the time I (Robert) met Jenny at the age of sixteen, neither of us can recall any earlier signs of bipolar disorder. It seemed to us the illness just came out of nowhere. From this point on, my life as a husband would change.

A good friend of mine, Pastor Mark Tossell, who himself has struggled with depression for thirty years, asked me once to describe what it is like being married to someone with serious, chronic depression. My one word response was "Challenging!"

I then went on to explain that at first we were both in the dark as to what was happening, so it became quite unnerving and challenging to recognise and understand why Jenny's mood swings became so erratic and her behaviour had changed. Once I understood the diagnosis it was a little easier to accept the inconsistencies that appeared in her behaviour.

Both manic and depressive episodes place incredible stress on the spouse, family and friends. Since people in a manic state can be unreasonable, emotional and impulsive, family members fear they will do something hurtful or disastrous. They may get the family into serious debt, have several affairs, quit their jobs and engage in other foolish behaviour. Family members of those in a depressed state can become extremely frustrated when, time after time, their efforts to support and encourage the sufferer are rejected and rebuffed.

Mental health has a way of cutting down our pride like no other illness can. For the one with the illness, pride does not seem to be an issue. They are either blissfully happy with the way they are and are unconcerned with what others think, or they are totally depressed about everything, or they are too confused to worry about pride. If they are concerned about what others think it is with suspicion, not embarrassment. But for those of us whose perceptions are not altered by these unique chemical imbalances, care-giving can be very humiliating when we are conscious of a stigma and what others may think. I have found that I needed to be constantly reminding myself that *"...we know that all things work together for good to them that love God, to them who are the called according to his purpose."* (Romans 8:28)

While the bipolar patient is going through an up or a down or a state of confusion, the spouse or care-giver is going through a shrinking of self. The first part of self that usually gets hit is pride. Our mentally-altered loved ones do not act in a 'socially acceptable' manner and we start to shrink. We love them enough to look beyond their differences; we still see them as unique and lovely, but we have to give up some of our pride to be with them, because our pride will make us afraid of what others might think. I got embarrassed and felt ashamed. It is so true what the Proverbs say *"The fear of man bringeth a snare: but whoso putteth his trust in the LORD shall be safe."* (Proverbs 29:25)

Mania can be very confusing to people and when your spouse ends up in a psychiatric ward, your embarrassment is coupled with shame. You prefer to avoid any discussion of it. Those who love you are also confused by it and they also might want to avoid raising the issue.

These were times when God was dealing with my pride. I would try to cover up another episode in case people may think it was impinging on my work abilities, or even that I may be the cause of her being in the state she was in.

As a pastor I came to a point of feeling hypocritical, as I would be preaching on trusting the Lord and not yielding to your fears and anxiety, knowing that my wife was at home lying in a bed sedated in order to sleep off another anxiety attack.

There were moments in my ministry life when I felt a complete failure. It was like I was hearing the words of Jesus warning what His scoffers and mockers had said to Him as He hung on the cross. *"And he said unto them, Ye will surely say unto me this proverb, **Physician, heal thyself**: whatsoever we have heard done in Capernaum, do also here in thy country."* (Luke 4:23)

I recently read a memoir by Neil Anderson in his book called "A Rough Road to Freedom". In the book he described his own journey trying to minister to others on freedom from bondages of anxiety, depression, fear and all types of addictions whilst his own wife was suffering through a sudden onset of a mental illness. He said "I was helping everyone else, but I couldn't help my wife, other than to just be there. I have always been known as 'mister fix-it.' Even my children would say, 'Don't worry, Dad will fix it.' But I couldn't fix this. I felt helpless."[21] He appropriately titled the chapter "Brokenness."

Part of my own issues were based in my faulty understanding of bipolar disorder. Foolishly and ignorantly I was like one of Job's miserable comforters, expecting and requesting Jenny to just "snap out of it." After all, didn't she realise she was ruining our family and my career! – How selfish I was!

Nowadays, after living with a spouse who has lived with the infirmity of bipolar depression for twenty three years, I have accepted her limitations and adjusted my expectations accordingly.

However, during the early stages of understanding Jenny's illness, it was difficult for me not to be selfish and expect way too much from her. I recall reading through the New Testament letter of Colossians and in particular a section that talks about the family roles and responsibilities. As I read the scripture the Lord rebuked me and helped me. One verse reads as follows: *"Husbands, love your wives,*

---

21 "A Rough Road to Freedom, Neil Anderson, Monarch Books, Grand Rapids, Michigan USA, 2012, page 169.

and be not bitter against them." *(Colossians 3:19)* Whilst I dearly loved my wife, I could see that I was becoming bitter and feeling as though I had been short-changed in life. This was a wake-up call from the Holy Spirit. I knew I needed to repent and change my attitude. Bipolar disorder was Jenny's sickness, but selfishness had become my illness. It was now time to literally fulfil the marriage vows that are often just repeated without fully understanding them - "I, Robert, take you, Jenny, to be my lawfully wedded wife, to have and to hold, from this day forward, for better, for worse, for richer, for poorer, in sickness and in health, until death do us part." It was the "in sickness" part that became my reality.

In 1998, we had the privilege of having evangelist Tom Williams from the USA visit our church to conduct a preaching and teaching series. I first heard of Dr Williams from a friend who recommended I listened to his testimony message called "Loving my wife back to health" and watched a movie about his life called "Twice Given".[22] He became known as 'America's preacher to those who are hurting.' He knew firsthand the sorrow that comes from the loss of a spouse and child. Later, he and his second wife, Pam, enjoyed a wonderful marriage for several years. Pam was an ideal wife and mother before being struck down with bacterial meningitis in 1978, leaving her with both physical and mental handicaps. As I listened to his story where he bared his heart as he told of the trials his family faced with Pam's illness, I was deeply challenged concerning the measure of my love for Jenny. Mrs Williams was in a coma for six weeks and the doctor told him that his wife was brain dead and could not live. He was advised to make the decision to pull the plugs and let her go, but he said, "Well, I don't feel like God wants me to do that." After eight weeks in two different hospitals, he took Mrs. Williams home in his arms, still in

---

22 A copy of the movie can be ordered online - http://www.twwm1.com/wordpress1/dvd/twice-given/

her comatose state. She was down to 38kg (84 pounds), her arms were in the foetal position and her legs turned in toward each other. Her feet turned down off her legs, her toes curled under her feet and her hands were deformed. One

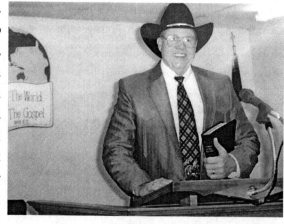

side of her face appeared like a stroke victim's face, her eyes and neck were locked. He began to do everything that he could for her at home that a registered nurse would have done. After six months of his caring for her, God woke her up one night. For over thirty years he loved her and cared for her as an invalid, mentally and physically.

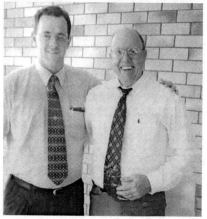

Top: Tom Williams;

Below: Robert with Dr Tom Williams in Rockhampton

He continued his evangelistic ministry, travelling all over the world and when possible he took Pam. For years on the airlines he carried her in his arms up and down narrow aisles to the bathroom. Mrs Williams went home to be with the Lord over ten years ago. God in His faithfulness used their experiences to change our lives.

Understanding my role as not only a husband but also at times the carer, has helped me to love my wife as myself during the trying times, knowing that God makes no mistakes. The life and testimony of Dr Williams helped me with this.

The apostle Peter gave some great advice as he was inspired by God to pen the third chapter of his first epistle. He gives us today some very clear instructions as a husband and a wife. The single quality that's talked about is a quality that's called 'submission.' When we hear that word, is our first feeling a positive one or a negative one? It's a little negative isn't it? In fact, 'submission' is not the kind of word we hear much about in the twenty-first century. It's one of those words that people think may be a little out of date. However, when you define the Bible word of 'submission', God is referring to having the courage to give up self rights to meet another person's needs. It is simply the ability to be unselfish in our relationships. This is exactly what I needed to hear in learning to live with a person suffering from bipolar disorder.

This ability to be unselfish in our relationships is one of the main ingredients to learning to live God's way. One section of 1 Peter gives step by step practical instructions for practicing unselfish living, *"Likewise, ye husbands, dwell with them according to knowledge, giving honour unto the wife, as unto the weaker vessel, and as being heirs together of the grace of life; that your prayers be not hindered. Finally, be ye all of one mind, having compassion one of another, love as brethren, be pitiful, be courteous:" (1 Peter 3:7-8)*

After reading passages like this and others, I began to realise how important it was for me to let Jenny know that my love for her is unconditional and never in question, even when I need to make difficult decisions in the process of her treatment. My wife needed to know that I understood what she was going through. I don't always get it right, but I do seek to follow the advice concerning my wife and *"...dwell with them according to knowledge, giving honour unto the wife, as unto the weaker vessel..."*

For me, unselfishness began when I started to ask, "What does Jenny need?" I needed to see that God had given me the role to honour and value her needs. If I know somebody's needs, I'm not going to begin to meet their needs unless I value them. I had to recognise that her needs, were as important as mine and to honour that value.

The challenge is not to be ready for the one big sacrifice and then it's back to my selfish ways. Rather, the challenge is to constantly make the little sacrifices of time, money, energy, ambitions, desires, plans and opportunities. Why? Because that's what love does!

The King James Bible uses a word to describe love in action or love with feet. It is the word "charity." This is what God requires of us in our submission to one another in our relationships. *"Charity suffereth long, and is kind; charity envieth not; charity vaunteth not itself, is not puffed up, Doth not behave itself unseemly, seeketh not her own, is not easily provoked, thinketh no evil; Rejoiceth not in iniquity, but rejoiceth in the truth; Beareth all things, believeth all things, hopeth all things, endureth all things."* (1 Corinthians 13:4-7)

PART 2

TRUTHS TO LIVE BY

CHAPTER 10

THE VOICE OF TRUTH

DELIVERANCE

The phrase "scientia est potentia" is a Latin aphorism meaning "knowledge is power". The origin of the phrase is commonly attributed to English philosopher, statesman, scientist and author, Sir Francis Bacon, who died in 1626. However, sixteen hundred years beforehand on the hills of Israel, a Jewish carpenter proclaimed the power of knowledge to set people free. Jesus Christ said, *"And ye shall know the truth, and the truth shall make you free." (John 8:32)*

Knowledge of the truth is the key to being set free from all forms of spiritual, mental and emotional bondage. In the same discourse by Jesus in John Chapter 8, He continues and warns of the devil's strategy to negate truth and keep people in captivity. *"Ye are of your father the devil, and the lusts of your father ye will do. He was a murderer from the beginning, and abode not in the truth, because there is no truth in him. When he speaketh a lie, he speaketh of his own: for he is a liar, and the father of it. And because I tell you the truth, ye believe me not." (John 8:44-45)*

Satan's greatest weapon is lies; Jesus' greatest weapon is truth. Life is literally a battle of lies versus truth. Depending on which we believe will determine whether we are set free from wrong thinking in our minds, or trapped. Bipolar can cause a person to have cognitive issues that make it difficult to discern between truth and lies. In fact a lie believed as truth, will affect your life as though it were true. For example, for many years, people did not believe that the world was round. They believed it was flat; and therefore, when they ventured out, they wouldn't go very far on the ocean, because they believed they might fall off the edge. That wasn't true, but because they believed the lie, it affected their lives as if it were true.

Growing up, I (Robert) recall one of my early primary school teachers telling me that if I crossed my eyes, and the wind changed or if I got hit in the head, my eyes would stay that way. That's not true, but I believed it and so I wouldn't even dare look at a fly on the end of my nose, or whatever, just in case it would happen.

When you believe a lie it hinders you from doing, accomplishing and experiencing all that God wants for your life. A lie believed as truth will affect your life. This is why the truth of God's Word and His promises must be known by a sufferer of bipolar so the lies often created through wrong thinking are dismissed.

Every lie is like a snare that can stop you in your tracks. The apostle Paul writes to tell us the devil loves to bind people in the snare of lies, but God's plan is to help people stay away from them. *"And that they may recover themselves out of the snare of the devil, who are taken captive by him at his will."* (2 Timothy 2:26)

Satan lies to us through deception. The enemy is the ultimate deceiver and, like a masterful illusionist using optical illusions to trick the eye, the devil uses lies to trick our minds. *"But I fear, lest by any means, as the serpent beguiled Eve through his subtilty, so your minds should be corrupted from the simplicity that is in Christ."* (2 Corinthians 11:3) He will take that which is evil and make it look good; that which is good and make it look evil. His desired outcome is confusion which plagues the mind of a Christian living with bipolar.

There are three common lies that our spiritual enemy will attack our minds with.

- Lie # 1 - *"My worth is determined by what I do and by what others think of me."* If I believe this lie, here's how it will affect my life: I'll become overly driven and become competitive. I will become so driven that I may sin, just to get to the bottom line or the final result. Oftentimes, I will become a workaholic. If I ever take time off, I'll feel guilty. Why? Because in my mind, my worth is determined by what I do or by what others think of me.

- Lie # 2 - *"I am the way I am and I can't change. This is just how I am. I can't overcome it."* If I believe this lie, it leads to passivity. It leads to shame. "I'm so ashamed of this, that I can't change." It leads to guilt. "If I were only better, I could overcome it, but since I can't, I feel guilty." Oftentimes, it will lead to resignation. "This is just how I am. I give up," All of a sudden, your relationships grow stale. Your purpose in life grows stale. Your contribution to others grows stale. "This is just the way I am. I can't change." It's a lie that, if believed as truth, will affect your life as though it were.

- Lie # 3 - *"If you really knew me, you wouldn't like me."* This leads us to a place of a living hypocrisy. We become actors. We try to convince people of something that we're not. Why? Deep down, we can never achieve true intimacy because in all reality, no one sees us as who we really are. The walls go up and no one's getting through these walls of protection. Those are some examples of the lies that we believe about ourselves. Are you bold enough to say, "Maybe it's one of these lies, or similar, but I'm believing and living something about myself that is not consistent with God's word. It's a lie."

Have you ever been caught off guard by not being able to recognise the voice on the other end of a telephone call? You listen intently to the sound and tone of the voice in an attempt to identify the caller. Then when you do recognise the voice there is a sense of relief, (unless you didn't want to be talking with them). The point is, you must be able to recognise the right voice.

In the world in which we live there are many voices calling for our mind's attention. Paul lets us know there are many languages in the world and they are all significant to someone, but not everyone. *"There are, it may be, so **many kinds of voices** in the world, and none of them is without signification. Therefore if I know not the meaning of the voice, I shall be unto him that speaketh a barbarian, and he that speaketh shall be a barbarian unto me." (1 Corinthians 14:10-11)*

When we talk about 'the voices in the world', we are not talking about hearing an audible voice in our head. Rather, we are referring to the thoughts and impressions we gain from the Bible, general literature, pondering, ideas, listening to media, church preaching, perceptions, people speaking to us and circumstances forming an opinion within us.

With the vulnerability of a bipolar-affected mind, the sufferer must constantly identify the voice he is listening to and ensure he is hearing the voice of truth not the voice of lies. Truth is the greatest source of deliverance from the lies one believes.

From a therapeutic standpoint, every person living with bipolar needs to know the truth of God and be able to discern His voice to avoid believing the devil's lies about their condition and future. The voice listened to will be the voice that determines success or failure. Knowing the truth and discerning the lies is the first step of any therapy for living with bipolar.

Many different voices will invade at once, seeking sufferers to follow their advice and ideas. The Christian must learn to discern through the noise and listen to the Lord: *"My sheep hear my voice, and I know them, and they follow me:" (John 10:27)*

There are various voices that want our attention: the voice of fear, the voice of failure, the voice of doubt, the voice of condemnation, the voice of false hope and many more. The voice of truth is different from the others and offers hope and deliverance from oppressive thoughts. Truth doesn't necessarily change the facts of your situation, but many times truth will ignore the facts. The facts say, "You can't walk on water." However truth says, "Peter, I am going to ignore that fact. Come unto me!" The facts say, "I have worked hard all week. I am tired." Truth says, "Come unto me, I will give you rest." Facts say, "My husband, my kids, my marriage, or my life is in serious trouble. Bipolar has crippled my future and I just don't see any way out." Truth says, "I am the way, the truth and the life." – Jesus is the Truth.

The Christian music group, Casting Crowns wrote a song entitled, "The Voice of Truth". They wrote lyrics aimed to encourage the listener to choose the right voice.

Oh, what I would do to have the kind of faith it takes
To climb out of this boat I'm in onto the crashing waves
To step out of my comfort zone into the realm of the unknown
Where Jesus is, and he's holding out his hand
But the waves are calling out my name and they laugh at me
Reminding me of all the times I've tried before and failed
The waves they keep on telling me time and time again
"Boy, you'll never win, you you'll never win"
But the Voice of truth tells me a different story
The Voice of truth says "do not be afraid!"
and the Voice of truth says "this is for My glory"

Out of all the voices calling out to me
I will choose to listen and believe the Voice of truth
Cause Jesus you are the Voice of truth
And I will listen to you.. oh you are the Voice of truth[23]

How can we know when God is speaking that we're not just listening to our own wishful thinking or deception? How do we know we are hearing the voice of truth? How do we know we're not just talking to ourselves? How do we know we're not confusing our own desires with the prompting of the Holy Spirit? There are three key steps to take to ensure we are following the voice of truth.

READ THE WORD OF GOD TO ENSURE YOUR DECISION IS CONSISTENT WITH IT.

"Sanctify them through thy truth: thy word is truth. As thou hast sent me into the world, even so have I also sent them into the world. And for their sakes I sanctify myself, that they also might be sanctified through the truth." (John 17:17-19)

The Bible is called 'the truth' and that is why one of the primary forms of therapy for a Christian with bipolar is to be reading and studying the Bible. The Word of God is the ultimate source of truth for mankind. The Bible needs to be the authority in matters, not my emotions or experiences.

The Bible is a unique book. It is a collection of 66 books written over a period of 1500 years by 40 different authors who were from 13 countries writing their contribution on 3 separate continents (Asia,

---

23 "Voice of Truth" is a song recorded by Casting Crowns and written by Mark Hall and Steven Curtis Chapman

Europe and Africa). From this book comes all the information that we have about God, Jesus, heaven, hell, salvation and eternity. It is the most powerful work of literature ever written; and Satan hates it!

The scriptures have the power within its pages to change us and reading it helps us to know what is right and what God requires of us. We will always know the thought we are having or 'voice' we are hearing in our heart is the voice of truth because it will always be consistent with the Word. It doesn't matter what the latest public opinion is. What matters is what God has to say to us. The voice of truth will equip you to know which path to take in life.

David said, *"Thy word is a lamp unto my feet, and a light unto my path." (Psalm 119:105)* In David's day there was limited night travel as there were no street lights. People wore ankle lights and held lanterns to help them see to take their next step. One couldn't see farther down the road, only how to make the next step. This is what the Bible does for us today. As you read the Word of God you are asking the Lord to show you your next step. The Word of God is a lamp to guide your feet and a light for your path. When you don't know which way to go, the Bible will tell you. When you don't know what to do, the Bible will tell you. When you don't know what to say, the Bible will tell you. When you don't know how to react, the Bible will tell you. God will never tell you to violate anything in His Word. God will never tell you to ignore or disobey anything in His book.

The Bible also gives us encouragement and hope. It lifts us up when we are down. It gives us strength when we are weak. It helps us to keep going when we want to quit.

RECEIVE THE WORD OF GOD EVEN WHEN YOUR DESIRES ARE IN CONFLICT WITH IT.

"For I know that in me (that is, in my flesh,) dwelleth no good thing: for to will is present with me; but how to perform that which is good I find not. For the good that I would I do not: but the evil which I would not, that I do. Now if I do that I would not, it is no more I that do it, but sin that dwelleth in me. I find then a law, that, when I would do good, evil is present with me. For I delight in the law of God after the inward man: But I see another law in my members, warring against the law of my mind, and bringing me into captivity to the law of sin which is in my members. O wretched man that I am! who shall deliver me from the body of this death? I thank God through Jesus Christ our Lord. So then with the mind I myself serve the law of God; but with the flesh the law of sin." (Romans 7:18-25)

You will never have victory until you realise there is part of you that has no good in it. That's your old nature. Paul was honest about it and he accepted his imperfections. He just realised the fact of life that when you're a Christian there are two natures in your being and life doesn't always go well. Living with bipolar is not sin, but the old nature can easily use your weakness to yield to its desires. We need to choose to follow the desires of God by yielding to the Word of God. Paul reminded us there is a battle for our mind taking place. Every good word, every good deed, every good thought, every good motive and every good thing is challenged by evil. If we are able to any good thing, it is always the result of a battle.

This old nature, the law of sin, drags you down like gravity. Paul said, "I feel trapped" and cried out in agony. "God, I can't change. I cannot change in my own power." Paul was at the end of his rope then he got a flash of hope, an answer, *"I thank God through Jesus Christ our Lord.*

So then with the mind I myself serve the law of God; but with the flesh the law of sin." (Romans 7:25) The fact is that living the Christian life without struggles is impossible. Paul's answer to winning this war was in choosing to listen to the voice of truth by receiving the word when it is preached, taught and read.

REST IN THE WORD OF GOD EVEN THOUGH YOUR DIRECTION IS CHALLENGED BY IT.

"So then faith cometh by hearing, and hearing by the word of God." *(Romans 10:17)*

When you hear the voice of truth it will provoke you to live by faith. You may think you are headed in one direction, then God steps in and directs your paths. *"Trust in the LORD with all thine heart; and lean not unto thine own understanding. In all thy ways acknowledge him, and he shall direct thy paths."* *(Proverbs 3:5-6)*

What then is Bible faith? It is not to believe in spite of evidence – that's superstition. It is not wishy-washy I believe it is possible' faith. It is not a 'hope so' feeling. It is a 'know so' confidence. Real faith acts and obeys. Faith is obeying God in spite of feelings, circumstances or consequences. Faith enables me to visualise the future in the present. Faith is seeing it in advance, being certain of what we do not see.

We must learn to perform what God wants us to do before we ever see the results. Sometimes we don't understand the why, but we have faith in the Who. We live by promises not explanations. Faith is obeying God when we don't understand, and it always involves taking a risk.

I (Jenny) found the most difficult aspect of having bipolar was when I felt out of control. During these times I needed to listen to the voice of truth and not panic. I needed to remind myself to rest in the Word of God and trust the Lord to direct my paths. He would lead me to the right people who at the right time were able to assist me with the appropriate treatment or course of action I needed.

At times everything inside me was telling me to run and flee to find a way of escape. I had to acknowledge these were not the voices of truth, but of lies. The Word of God instructed me to rest, wait, acknowledge the Lord, pray, seek His face and come before His presence with thanksgiving. However, the last thing I wanted to do was to thank God for what was happening to me. But the voice of truth reminded me this was all for His glory and to thank Him even when I didn't understand. Every time God tells you to do something, it's a test. It's a test of whom I am going to believe - God or my gut.

Faith is believing God is doing something right now, even though I don't see it. One of the most comforting thoughts for those living with bipolar is that God is always at work in our lives. The answer is already on its way: He's moving the pieces into place even as you read this book. The voice of truth gives you a great peace – that's why you can rest in His Word.

What you discover in life often depends on what you are listening for. If you are listening for truth you can discern it and live by it. However, if you are not listening for it, you may very well miss the voice of truth and be deceived by a lie. An American Indian was walking in downtown New York City alongside a friend who was a resident of the city. Right in the centre of Manhattan, the Indian seized his friend's arm and whispered, "Wait! I hear a cricket." His friend said, "Come on! A cricket? Man, this is downtown New York." He persisted, "No, seriously, I really do." "It's impossible!" was the response. "You can't hear a cricket with the taxis going by, car horns honking, people screaming at each other and brakes screeching." Both sides of the street were filled with people. Cash registers were clanging in the background and the subway was roaring beneath. "You can't possibly hear a cricket". The Indian insisted, "Wait a minute" He led his friend along, slowly. They stopped and the Indian walked to the end of the block, crossed the street, looked around, then cocked his head to one side. He crossed another street and there in a large cement planter a tree was growing. He dug into the mulch and found the cricket. "See!" he yelled, as he held the insect high above his head. His friend marvelled and asked, "How in the world could it be that you heard a cricket in the middle of busy downtown Manhattan?" The Indian said, "Well, my ears are different from yours. It simply depends on what you're listening for. Here, let me show you." He reached in his pocket and pulled out a handful of change - a couple of quarters, three or four nickels and some dimes and pennies. Then he said, "Now watch." He held the coins waist high and dropped them to the sidewalk. Every head within a block turned around and looked in the direction of the Indian. It all depends on what you're listening for!

CHAPTER 11

RIGHT THINKING MAKES A DIFFERENCE

DELIBERATIONS

A n entry in a wife's diary read as follows:

Tonight I thought my husband was acting weird. We had made plans to meet at a nice restaurant for dinner. I was shopping with my friends all day long, so I thought he was upset at the fact that I was a bit late, but he made no comment on it. Conversation wasn't flowing, so I suggested that we go somewhere quiet so we could talk. He agreed, but he didn't say much. I asked him what was wrong. He said, "Nothing." I asked him if it was my fault that he was upset. He said he wasn't upset, that it had nothing to do with me and not to worry about it. On the way home, I told him that I loved him. He smiled slightly and kept driving. I can't explain his behaviour I don't know why he didn't reply, "I love you, too." When we got home, I felt as if I had lost him completely, as if he wanted nothing to do with me anymore. He just sat there quietly and watched TV. He continued to seem distant and absent. Finally, with silence all around us, I decided to go to bed. About 15 minutes later, he came to bed. But I still felt that he was distracted and his thoughts were somewhere else. He fell asleep; I cried. I don't know what to do. *I'm almost sure that his thoughts are with someone else. My life is a disaster.*

The same day an entry in the husband's diary read as follows:

A four putt! Who four putts in golf from two feet away from hole? Arghhh!

Our thinking gets us all messed up at times, especially negative thinking. At times as a pastor I (Robert) have thoughts like, "I am completely fried. I don't know if I can do this for another day. Who knows if I'm even making a difference anyway? I wonder if they really even care. Will this sermon be any good, anyway? I mean, what do I have to offer? Maybe it's just too much for me." Every now and then I need to take an attitude check. The problem for me is, it's all in my head.

Thoughts get scrambled during moments of bipolar; I (Jenny) recognise this fact. There will be times when all I can focus on is the negative and bad things, at other times during a high moment, my thoughts are elated and only positive and grandiose. It's not the thinking pattern that triggers a bipolar episode, rather, it is often the result of a bipolar episode. While there may be times when negative thinking can spiral a person into depression, it is not always the case with a person suffering from bipolar. Rather, it is the onset of a depressive episode that can bring about negative thought patterns. I have never thought myself into a bipolar depression nor have I ever thought myself into a manic moment; these states of mind just happen and then my thinking is affected.

The only difference between Robert's and my thought-patterns is that bipolar tends to create an environment in my mind conducive to the creation of extreme thoughts. This is why I need to constantly capture my thoughts and ensure I'm not allowing my illness to carry me away into wrong thinking. The Bible puts it this way, *"For though we walk in the flesh, we do not war after the flesh: (For the weapons of our warfare are not carnal, but mighty through God to the **pulling down of strong holds**;) Casting down imaginations, and every high thing that exalteth itself against the knowledge of God, and **bringing into captivity every thought to the obedience of Christ**; And having in a readiness to revenge all disobedience, when your obedience is fulfilled."* (2 Corinthians 10:3-6)

Strongholds were places of fortification and security used for military advantage. *"And the hand of Midian prevailed against Israel: and because of the Midianites the children of Israel made them the dens which are in the mountains, and caves, and **strong holds**."* (Judges 6:2)

The apostle Paul uses this analogy but likens our wrong thoughts as strongholds that gain the advantage over us. These must be pulled down through right thinking.

Another aspect of a stronghold is that they are not out in the open or easily exposed. *"And David went up from thence, and dwelt in **strong holds** at Engedi."* (1 Samuel 23:29) You may have some negative strongholds that shape your thinking that you are not even aware of. A strong hold has a STRONG HOLD on you. You are a prisoner locked by deception. A stronghold is well defended and difficult to attack.

Let me illustrate a stronghold this way. Have you seen those little electric invisible dog gates or fences. Depending where you place the little beam, the poor little unsuspecting dog moves toward it and what happens when he crosses the barrier? He gets zapped! When the dog gets zapped enough, what will he do? He'll stop trying to get out! You can turn the switch off. The electric fence is not even on and the dog will never cross that line. Why? Because in his mind, he is a prisoner locked by this barrier. That's a stronghold.

Have you ever been to a circus and seen a giant elephant with a small rope around its ankle? Did you ever stop to think, hey, wait a minute? Physically speaking, there is no way that small little rope can hold back that giant elephant! And did you ever wonder how it happened that a giant elephant could be held in place by something that does not have the power to contain him. Here's how it works. When trainers begin taming a baby elephant, they place a heavy chain around its ankle and stake the chain into the ground. Day after day, hour after hour, the baby elephant struggles to escape. But his efforts are in vain. He simply cannot break free from the grips of that powerful chain. Eventually he surrenders. He resolves in his mind that there is no possible way he can escape that chain. So he relinquishes forever the struggle to be free. Then when he has given up trying, his masters replace that giant chain with the small rope. If the elephant ever opened his eyes to the truth, he could break free at any moment. All it would take is one try, but since the elephant doesn't know that, he doesn't take a step in the right direction of freedom. And so it happens that ten, twenty, thirty years later, the giant elephant remains held in bondage by something that really has no power to control him, except the power he chooses to give it. That's a stronghold.

Some people have strongholds in their mind and their thoughts go like this:

- "I can never go beyond this point."
- "I will always have negative thoughts, I can't help it."
- "I can never have a good relationship with my spouse."
- "I can never have an intimate relationship with God."

- "I could never be good enough."
- "I could never have a good relationship with other people."
- "I could never change. I will never be anything but bipolar"
- "I will never be anything but addicted. This is just the way I am."
- "I will never be able to forgive."

That's a stronghold.

Satan's strongholds are thoughts. If the devil can get you to entertain his thoughts such as fear, anxiety, doubt, apprehension and so on, he can have a doorway to controlling your mind. He will put a ring in your nose and lead you around, if you let him. But, we don't have to let him.

The Word of God tells us how to be victorious and shows us how to be more than conquerors in Him who loved us and gave Himself for us. We do not overcome strongholds with the weapons of this world; but instead, with the weapons of God. God is able to overthrow the strongholds. *"Thou hast broken down all his hedges; thou hast brought his strong holds to ruin." (Psalm 89:40)*

We demolish strongholds with God's truth. We take captive every thought and when the thought doesn't line up with truth – "Chuck it out!" What do we do with it? We make it obedient to Christ. We cast down everything that is not of God and we take it captive. Rather than us being the prisoner of the stronghold, we take the lie as our prisoner, then we make it obedient to Christ. We let the power of God change our thinking. This is called renewing our mind.

We cast down strongholds by renewing our mind. *"I beseech you therefore, brethren, by the mercies of God, that ye present your bodies* *a living sacrifice, holy, acceptable unto God, which is your reasonable service. And be not conformed to this world: but **be ye transformed by the renewing of your mind**, that ye may prove what is that good, and acceptable, and perfect, will of God." (Romans 12:1-2)*

We are also instructed further to *"be **renewed** in the spirit of your mind;" (Ephesians 4:23)*

How do we recognise a renewed mind? How should we be thinking? Again we turn to the authority for life, the Word of God. The apostle Paul exhorts us to adopt a mind like Jesus. I need to renew my thinking – to think as the Lord Jesus thinks. *"Let this mind be in you, which was also in Christ Jesus:" (Philippians 2:5)*

The Bible says our mind or attitude should be the same as that of Christ Jesus. We see what Jesus endured for us. He suffered and died for us, only living to glorify God, yet He never complained. We cannot find one example in scripture where Jesus reflected a negative attitude. Our attitude should be the same as that of Christ Jesus.

'In His Steps' is a best-selling religious fiction novel written by Charles Monroe Sheldon. It was first published in 1896 and has sold more than 30,000,000 copies. The full title of the book is 'In His Steps: What Would Jesus Do?' Flowing on from this the acrostic WWJD from the subtitle 'What would Jesus do' has served as a good reminder to people to think about their actions. But prior to that we need to ask – WWJT? – What would Jesus think?

If I (Jenny) can guard my thoughts, especially during a bipolar episode, it is extremely helpful in maintaining a balanced mind when my brain chemicals are screaming "go radical."

There are clear characteristics of the mind of Christ in the second chapter of Philippians.

A Mind of Selflessness – *"Who, being in the form of God, thought it not robbery to be equal with God: But made himself of no reputation,…"* (Philippians 2:6-7a)

He was God, yet He made himself of no reputation in contrast to the quest of many to "climb the ladder of success" and make a name for themselves.

A Mind of Service – *"… and took upon him the form of a servant, and was made in the likeness of men:"* (Philippians 2:7b)

Jesus became a servant for us. In a world where everyone is climbing the ladder of success, there is not much competition for the bottom rung. Too many people spell service – "Serve us".

A Mind of Submission – *"And being found in fashion as a man, he humbled himself, and became obedient unto death, even the death of the cross."* (Philippians 2:8)

Are you willing to do anything God asks? Is there anything that you are unwilling to do? What an incredible mindset and attitude – the mind of Christ.

Our decisions, our thought processes, our mental state and our attitudes should be like those of Christ Jesus.

When our only daughter, Anna, was growing up at home we'd sometimes call her 'Anna – mated'. She was animated at times. When she was about seven years old I (Robert) had returned from a trip to the United States of America bringing her a toy 'Piglet' from the Disney program 'Winnie the Pooh'. We were driving down the road

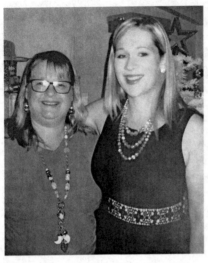
Jenny with Anna

one day when Anna frantically cried out from the back seat, "Stop, stop, something really bad has just happened." Jenny and I wondered what had happened. What did she see? a dead animal? a dead person? a car wreck, or whatever? To our surprise the crisis was 'Piglet' just fell out the window. She had wanted to give him some air and was holding him out the window when he slipped from her hand. Our little girl was distraught, so as a father of 'daddy's little girl', I dutifully turned the car around to go back and search for 'Piglet' on the side of the road. We never found 'Piglet', which turned Anna from distraught to despairing.

That kind of attitude is a reflection of what we often have. We take something that's not that big of a deal and we make it a big deal. We don't lose Piglet – we lose the remote control, or the keys, or the phone, or a letter, or misplace an item. We take something that is slightly negative and let it grow into an enormous battle in our minds. Yet, we are to have the mind of Christ. Our thought process and our decisions should be as those of Christ Jesus. We need to renew our thinking and this is particularly important for bipolar sufferers.

IDENTIFY YOUR NEGATIVE THOUGHT PATTERNS

Most of us battle with negative thoughts in different ways and we need to *"take heed"* to what we do: *"Wherefore let him that thinketh he standeth take heed lest he fall." (1 Corinthians 10:12)* Take a brief examination and identify areas of negativity in your thinking. Place a ✓ in the box or boxes that you identify with.

❑ **Personal Negativity** – Are you negative about things about yourself? Do you think thoughts like: "I don't have what it takes, you know, I can't do it all. No matter how hard I try, I can't get it all done." "Everyone else gets all the breaks, not me." "No one appreciates me, I just give and give and give." "No one knows just how valuable I am." Maybe personal negativity for you has to do with your physical body: "If I could just take a little bit of this and move it to somewhere else. You know, that would be great." Some men might think, "If only the hair on my head would grow half as fast as the hair in my ears, wouldn't that be a great day?"

❑ **People Negativity** – Are you negative about your relationships? Do you think thoughts like: "Every time I trust a person, I get burned." "You can't trust men as far as you can throw 'em. They're all the same." "Oh, I wish that my wife was like so and so." "I wish that my husband was different, if I have to pick up another pair of his dirty underwear…" "He'll never change." "She'll never change." Maybe your relational negativity has to do with work: "My boss is a fool and I can't stand working with all these people" Maybe your negativity has to do with family members. "Everything is so messed up in my family."

❑ **Positional Negativity** – Are you negative because of the circumstances in your life? Singles think: "If I were married, then I'd be happy." Married people think: "If I were married to somebody else, then I'd be happy." "If we only had children, then we'd be happy." "If we only had different children, then we'd be happy." Working people think: "If I had a better job." "If I had more money." "If I had a car that worked." "If I had a bigger house." "I'll never get out of debt. Life is not fair." "Circumstances get me down." Are you negative about your position in life?

☐ **Pious Negativity** – Are you negative in your stance on spiritual issues? Do you think thoughts like: "Why is it that God answers everybody else's prayers, but when I pray nothing seems to happen?" "Never do business with Christians – they are all crooks." Do you get spiritual negativity towards churches? "There's not a church in town that lives up to my standards." Spiritual negativity thinks along the lines of: "How come I can't get close to God?" "All I can find in the Bible are verses with negative connotations."

☐ **Picky Negativity** – This is a kind of a catchall negative thinking where you get very nit-picky toward everyone and anything. For example, you're driving the car and someone is going incredibly slow in front of you and that just makes you crazy. You don't swear, but you want to, and when you scream past them, you think "Amen!" You get annoyed about little things that in the scheme of things don't really matter. You think thoughts like: "Why don't they hire someone who speaks English?" "My hair won't do what I want it to."

Before we can defeat a negative thought pattern, we must identify that it's there and be willing to change. Some people never defeat a negative thought pattern because they decide to be miserable and are intent on finding negativity. If we want to find things to whinge about we'll find them. If we want to find things to be upset about, we'll find them.

Think of two birds - a vulture and a hummingbird. What does a vulture find? A vulture finds dead things. What does a hummingbird find? Flowers, nectar and sweet things. Why do they find these things? Because they will find what they are looking for. If a person wants to find dead things, negative things, things to whinge and complain about, he will find them. However, if you want to find God's presence, His goodness, you can find those as well. It's all in your thinking.

Our minds have their own perceptions of life, that's why we need new thinking. No matter who or what has left an impression upon us, God's Word prevails. The key to changing our life is to change the way we think. The scripture teaches that the way we think determines the way we feel and the way we feel determines the way we act. Most people try to change themselves by changing the way they feel or the way they act, rather than going to the source and changing the way they think. We cannot change the way we feel. Feelings don't respond well to command. Feelings cannot be controlled. But the source of feelings can, and that is how we think.

Thinking affects who we are. Whatever we think about, we will become like that. *"For as he thinketh in his heart, so is he:..." (Proverbs 23:7)* We will become that which we think.

In 1979 Bob Geldof from the Rock band Boomtown Rats read a report on the shooting spree of 16-year-old Brenda Spencer, who fired at children playing in a school playground at Cleveland Elementary School in San Diego, on 29th January 1979. She killed two adults and injured eight children and one police officer. Spencer showed no remorse for her crime and her full explanation for her actions was, "I don't like Mondays; this livens up the day." Geldof wrote the song: "I don't like Mondays, Tell me why, I don't like Mondays, I wanna shoot the whole day down".

The Bible says God made Mondays – *"This is the day which the LORD hath made; we will rejoice and be glad in it." (Psalm 118:24)* Mondays are from God, they're His day and there is no reason why I have to just accept it as a bad day. Instead, I can make a Biblical choice to focus my attitude, not on what has been, but instead on what could be. This is God's day and if it's God's day, there is no reason why I have to make it a bad day.

ISOLATE THE SOURCES OF NEGATIVITY

There are two areas that will help you overcome and isolate yourself from negativity.

Avoid spending time with negative people – *"Be not deceived: evil communications corrupt good manners." (1 Corinthians 15:33); "He that walketh with wise men shall be wise: but a companion of fools shall be destroyed." (Proverbs 13:20)* Bad company will corrupt good character. During 'low' moments in my illness, I (Jenny) only want people in my inner circle who will draw me closer to God and help with my thinking.

Abstain from dwelling on negative thoughts – *"Wherefore **gird up the loins of your mind**, be sober, and hope to the end for the grace that is to be brought unto you at the revelation of Jesus Christ;" (1 Peter 1:13)* We have to make a conscious effort not to dwell on negative thoughts. They may enter our mind, but we cannot let them stay there and fester.

We must then take a third step of action.

Actively replace negative thoughts with God's thoughts – *"Thou wilt keep him in perfect peace, whose mind is stayed on thee: because he trusteth in thee." (Isaiah 26:3)* Instead of, "My spouse will never change," maybe, "God is going to change me." Instead of, "I'll never climb out of debt," think, "With God, all things are possible." Instead of, "I'm not good enough and I can't," think, "I can do all things through Christ which strengtheneth me." Instead of, "I'm always gonna be the victim," think, "I am an overcomer." By the blood of the Lamb and by the words of our testimony, we replace negative thoughts with God's thoughts.

We must be renewed with truth from the Word of God. We are not transformed by good works, by religious activity or by external effort. We are transformed by the renewing of our minds. When we receive the truth we are spiritually and supernaturally changed by rejecting that which is not of God and embracing that which is of God.

Consider some of the common lies we can easily embrace when in bipolar moments:

- **Lie** – "God has left me."

    Truth – *"Let your conversation be without covetousness; and be content with such things as ye have: for he hath said, I will never leave thee, nor forsake thee." (Hebrews 13:5)*

- **Lie** – "No good will come of this."

    Truth – *"And we know that all things work together for good to them that love God, to them who are the called according to his purpose."(Romans 8:28)*

- **Lie** – "People hurt me."

Truth – *"For we wrestle not against flesh and blood, but against principalities, against powers, against the rulers of the darkness of this world, against spiritual wickedness in high places."(Ephesians 6:12)*

* **Lie** – "God is punishing me."

  Truth – *"For whom the Lord loveth he chasteneth, and scourgeth every son whom he receiveth"(Hebrews 12:6)*

* **Lie** – "I am weak."

  Truth – *"And he said unto me, My grace is sufficient for thee: for my strength is made perfect in weakness. Most gladly therefore will I rather glory in my infirmities, that the power of Christ may rest upon me."(2 Corinthians 12:9)*

* **Lie** - "I'll never make it."

  Truth - *"I can do all things through Christ which strengtheneth me."(Philippians 4:13)*

* **Lie** – "I am a victim."

  Truth – *"Nay, in all these things we are more than conquerors through him that loved us."(Romans 8:37)*

INVITE THE RIGHT THOUGHTS INTO YOUR MIND

We can renew our minds by inviting the right thoughts into our minds and choosing the areas to think upon. God gives us a list, *"Finally, brethren, whatsoever things are true, whatsoever things are honest, whatsoever things are just, whatsoever things are pure, whatsoever things are lovely, whatsoever things are of good report; if there be any virtue, and if there be any praise, think on these things."* (*Philippians 4:8*) If you are experiencing trouble with your thought life, don't overcome it by not thinking about the problem. Instead you need to do what God says – refocus. Attention creates access, so if negative thoughts have access into your mind it is because you have given those thoughts your attention.

Try right now to not think about something. Don't think about ice cream, don't think about vanilla ice cream with chocolate topping, don't think about ice cream. Most people immediately visualise what they are trying not to think about.

God gives us eight things to refocus on:

- Things that are **true** - Truth is found in the Word.

- Things that are **honest** - Honest conversations and dealings of men.

- Things that are **just** - God's ways are always just.

- Things that are **pure** - We need to ask God to cleanse our mind from sin.

- Things that are **lovely** - Jesus is altogether lovely – *Song of Solomon 5:16*

- Things that are of **good report** - We need to look for what is best in people.

- If there is any **virtue** in thinking on any of these things, then think on them. Virtue is moral excellence, goodness, God's greatness.

- Things that are of any **praise** - Think about what God is doing that is worth praising.

Ask God to replace the negative lies of this world with His truth and renew your mind. Thank Him for His blessings in your life and His goodness. Thank Him by faith for the great relationships He's given you. Thank Him by faith that He is here right now, that He is transforming your life. Thank Him by faith that your life will never be the same, because you are not going to have the negative attitudes of this world. Change starts in your mind – It's all in your head.

Victor Frankl, a survivor of the Nazi Holocaust, made an amazing statement of his formula for surviving the impossible years in the death camps. "Everything can be taken from us but one thing: the last of human freedoms - to choose one's attitude in any given set of circumstances."

Chris Carrier of Coral Gables, Florida, was abducted when he was 10 years old. His kidnapper, angry with the boy's family, burned him with cigarettes, stabbed him numerous times with an ice pick, then shot him in the head and left him to die in the Everglades. Remarkably, the boy survived, though he lost sight in one eye. No one was ever arrested. In 1997, a man confessed to the crime. Carrier, now a youth minister at Granada Presbyterian Church, went to see him with a trusted pastor friend. They found David McAllister, a 77-year-old ex-convict, frail and blind, living in a nursing home. In Chris's own words: *"It was awkward. What do you say to someone who'd tried to kill you? At first, McAllister denied trying to kill me. But as the pastor questioned him gently, he admitted he had left me there in the Everglades. He then held my hand and apologised for what he had done. I told him that I had forgiven him."* He returned almost everyday to visit David, introducing him to his wife and two girls. He shared the gospel with him and he (David) trusted in Christ. David

McAllister died 3 weeks later. The only people at his graveside funeral service were Chris Carrier, Chris's wife and their two daughters. After 22 years, the statute of limitations on the crime is long past. When asked if he felt the desire to seek revenge against McAllister, Carrier said, *"While many people can't understand how I could forgive David McAllister, from my point of view I couldn't not forgive him. If I'd chosen to hate him all these years, or spent my life looking for revenge, then I wouldn't be the man I am today, the man my wife and children love, the man God has helped me to be."*

That's what we call renewing our thinking to be like Jesus.

CHAPTER 12

BIPOLAR SAYS … BUT HOPE REPLIES

DISCERNMENT

On 5 January 1997, in the Antarctic Ocean south of Australia, British yachtsman Tony Bullimore's yacht, Exide Challenger capsized. The keel snapped in half. He was able to find an air pocket in the hull of the boat and survived. He was rescued by the Australian Navy after four days in freezing conditions. He admitted he had almost given up hope when a diver banged on the side of his boat. He started shouting: "I'm coming, I'm coming." It took a few seconds to get from one end of the boat to the other. Then he took a few deep breaths and dived out of the boat. They asked him where he found the hope to hang on for four days. He said, "I prayed and ate chocolate!"

There is a tremendous power in hope that enables us to go on despite the opposing conditions. Hope affects our emotions and affects our attitude. A hope in the future gives you strength in the present problem.

But, what happens when we lose hope? Have you ever been in a situation where you lost hope? I (Jenny) have, during the darkness of despair in a depression episode. In those moments faith wanes because hope has faded. The Bible mentions the connection between faith and hope. You cannot have faith unless you have hope. *"Now faith is* the substance of things *hoped for,* the evidence of things not seen." *(Hebrews 11:1)*

If we personified bipolar we could argue that it has the ability to rob life of hope, just like the Grinch who stole Christmas. Unfortunately, unlike in the Dr Seuss fable where, following an epiphany, the redeemed Grinch starts a new life with the Whos, commemorating the Christmas feast with them in his cave, bipolar doesn't change. It always seeks to deplete the sufferer of hope.

Words can make a big difference in giving or taking hope. When our firstborn son, Ben, was just under two years old, we noticed a lump on his chest that continued to grow in size. After some testing by our family doctor, he referred us to a surgeon to have the lump removed and to determine if it was malignant or benign. As they wheeled our little boy away into theatre we prayed and were anxiously waiting for news from the surgeon. His words had the power to dramatically affect our hope. If the words from his lips were, "Everything was very successful", our hope of full recovery would soar. If, however, his demeanour matched a sombre tone while uttering, "There have been some complications" then our hope would be depleted. Thankfully he gave us good news: the lump was benign and all was well. Hope soared!

Words can alter our hope in an instant. The words that Jeremiah the prophet heard and remembered infused him with hope. This in turn gave him strength to endure the sad and tragic moment of the destruction of his beloved city Jerusalem. *"And I said, My strength and **my hope is perished** from the LORD: Remembering mine affliction and my misery, the wormwood and the gall. My soul hath them still in remembrance, and is humbled in me. **This I recall to my mind, therefore have I hope.** It is of the LORD'S mercies that we are not consumed, because his compassions fail not." (Lamentations 3:18-*

22) He was able to refocus his thoughts to a promise of God which enabled him to resolve: "I can go on now". Hope came.

The Bible is a book full of hope for the believer. In referring to the Word of God, the apostle Paul said, *"For whatsoever things were written aforetime were written for our learning, that we through patience and comfort of the scriptures might have hope." (Romans 15:4)*

When life hurts and dreams fail, we need to hope in God's power, promises and protection. When we're trapped in a tunnel of misery, hope points to the light at the end. When we're overworked and exhausted, hope gives fresh energy to go on. When we're discouraged, hope in God lifts our spirit. When we are tempted to quit, hope keeps us going. When we lose our way and confusion blurs our vision and destination, hope dulls the edge of panic. When we struggle with a crippling disease, hope helps us live beyond the pain. When we fear the worst, hope renews our anticipation. When we find ourselves unemployed, hope encourages us to start over. When we must endure the consequences of a bad decision, hope fuels our recovery. When we say farewell to a saved loved one, hope gets us through the grieving. When we have a mental illness, like bipolar, hope in the Lord enables us to live with purpose.

During World War II several Australians were captured in Singapore by the Japanese and held in harsh conditions in Prisoner of War camps. Soldiers from many allied forces were captives together and several lost hope, sanity and their lives. However, when the war ended and the Japanese surrendered in 1945, the first allied flag to be raised in Singapore was an Australian flag. The Aussie prisoners maintained their hope for freedom and had made the flag in secret waiting for their liberation day.

Without hope people are in despair, destruction and depression. Without hope students get discouraged and drop out. Without hope athletes fall into a slump. Without hope addicts return to their habits. Without hope spouses decide to divorce. Without hope businessmen lose their drive and creativity. Hope in God is essential to life and especially to those suffering from a mental illness.

Nobody would disagree that bipolar disorder brings its fair share of trauma and pain, not necessarily physical but emotional and mental anguish and torment. Some have described the episodes of bipolar like a pregnant woman enduring her discomfort and pangs waiting to be delivered from her pain. Who can outdo the descriptive powers of a pregnant woman trying to explain her discomfort to the uninitiated? Words like "daggers", "twisting", "wringing" and "bloating" have never been used to such graphic extent. All this comes before she goes into labour! How do doctors, nurses, husbands and other family and friends help these women endure the pain? They try to keep them focused on the joy to come – the birth of the child. Jesus said *"A woman when she is in travail hath sorrow, because her hour is come: but as soon as she is delivered of the child, she remembereth no more the anguish, for joy that a man is born into the world." (John 16:21)*

The Bible describes the suffering of this world in a similar way. We've all had agony in life. We've all been pierced by the daggers of loss and disappointment. As a woman suffering with bipolar I (Jenny) can testify to the pain that accompanies the times of the vacillating highs and lows. For those believers who suffer with bipolar disorder, there are some words of hope recorded by the apostle Paul in the eighth chapter of the book of Romans. He reminds us that at the end of our labours are a glory and a joy so great that our pains won't even be remembered. As a Christian I can have an eternal perspective, not just a temporal view of life. No matter what happens in life, no matter what trials, there is hope. No situation is hopeless if you have the Holy Spirit in your life. That's what Romans 8:18-27 talks about. What is it that makes you strong enough to handle problems and difficulties of life? Paul says it is 'hope', and uses that word six times in these ten verses of scripture. Hope comes from having the right perspective.

Bipolar is going to say many things to you, but hope replies.

BIPOLAR SAYS: "IT'S NEVER GOING TO END." HOPE REPLIES: "IT WILL CEASE!"

"For I reckon that the sufferings of this present time are not worthy to be compared with the glory which shall be revealed in us. For the earnest expectation of the creature waiteth for the manifestation of the sons of God. For the creature was made subject to vanity, not willingly, but by reason of him who hath subjected the same in hope, Because the creature itself also shall be delivered from the bondage of corruption into the glorious liberty of the children of God. For we know that the whole creation groaneth and travaileth in pain together until now." (Romans 8:18-22)

The key to suffering is all in the way you look at it. Your problem is not the actual problem. Your problem is the way you look at your problem. Pauls says, "In my opinion whatever we may have to go through now is less than nothing compared with the magnificent future God has planned for us." The fact is, when I'm in pain I'm usually pretty short-sighted. I'm hurting. I'm not in the mood for long range planning. When you're in pain, what do you tend to look at? Your pain, your dilemma because of bipolar. That's all you see. That's all you feel. All you see is yourself. The biggest temptation when we're going through a problem is we focus on ourselves. "I don't see anybody else. All I see is me." Paul says, "That's your problem. You've got a short vision."

In these few verses God gives us His replies to life's perspective. We ought to look beyond our pain and see other things that will help us make it through our problem. That will give us hope and hope is what we need to make it.

In his autobiography, *Doctor's Progress*, American cardiologist, Dr Wilson McNair, said, "Hope is the medicine I use more than any other. Hope can cure nearly everything...There is an increasing body of medical evidence to support that idea that hope fosters health both physically and emotionally. But as soon as we lose hope there is not much chance things will change for the better." Psychiatrists have long suspected that hope fosters health both physically and emotionally.[24] There is an increasing body of medical evidence that documents the affect that depression and hopelessness have on physical health.[25]

Paul reminds us of a fundamental truth of the Christian life. We are not home yet. *"For I reckon that the sufferings of this present time are not worthy to be compared with the glory which shall be revealed in us." (Romans 8:18)* While we wait to be delivered from this world, we need to remember that we are living in a world that is under a curse. As a result of that curse, there is a lot of groaning and turmoil taking place. In the midst of all that, it is easy to become discouraged and it is easy to want to give up. The first thing Paul says about suffering

---

24 Relationship between hopelessness and ultimate suicide: a replication with psychiatric outpatients. Beck AT, Brown G, Berchick RJ, Stewart BL, Steer RA; Am J Psychiatry. 1990 Feb; 147(2):190-5.
25 The effect of depression treatment on elderly patients' preferences for life-sustaining medical therapy. *Ganzini L, Lee MA, Heintz RT, Bloom JD, Fenn DS; Am J Psychiatry. 1994 Nov; 151(11):1631-6.*

that will give us hope is that it is only temporary. We have a hope that we can look for. We have a hope that we know, no matter what we're going through, it's temporary. Even if I live with bipolar my entire life, that's nothing compared to the millions of years I'll be spending with the Lord. Paul points out there is no comparison between our present suffering and our future glory. Thank God, everything in this life is temporary, but Jesus is coming again! When Jesus Christ comes back everything is going to be set right. That's something we can put our hope in. Whatever happens to us now can never compare to what God has in store for us. There is no bipolar in Heaven! God has great things in store for us. *"But as it is written, Eye hath not seen, nor ear heard, neither have entered into the heart of man, the things which God hath prepared for them that love him."* (1 Corinthians 2:9)

BIPOLAR SAYS: "IT WILL ALWAYS BE LIKE THIS." HOPE REPLIES: "THINGS WILL CHANGE!"

"And not only they, but ourselves also, which have the firstfruits of the Spirit, even we ourselves groan within ourselves, waiting for the adoption, to wit, the redemption of our body. For we are saved by hope: but hope that is seen is not hope: for what a man seeth, why doth he yet hope for? But if we hope for that we see not, then do we with patience wait for it." (Romans 8:23-25)

If you are a born again Christian, there has been an inward change but the outside is still the same. However, there is an outward change coming one day: *"the redemption of our body"*. When Paul says *"we are saved by hope"*, the hope has nothing to do with the salvation of the soul. The context is the salvation of the physical body. Remember it is possibly the malfunctions in the brain, a physical organ of the body, that potentially causes bipolar. Thankfully, our present sinful body will be changed at the rapture of the church when Jesus comes again. Paul calls the rapture our *"blessed hope"* because that's when we get our glorified body and brain. *"Looking for that blessed hope, and the glorious appearing of the great God and our Saviour Jesus Christ."* *(Titus 2:13)* When we get to heaven, we are trading this old body in on a new, improved model! All the aches, pains and things that don't work right will be replaced. That's something I can put my hope in.

One day we'll be with the Lord and we'll have a perfect body. When we get our glorified body, salvation is finally completed. Hope is the anticipation and expectation in the heart of the believer for the imminent return of Jesus. We have no doubt that He is coming, we just don't know when. Since the rapture hasn't taken place, we wait. It is still a hope for us until then. That is why hope that is seen is not hope. If Jesus had already returned then our hope would be fulfilled: Hope would be History!

BIPOLAR SAYS: "NOBODY REALLY CARES." HOPE REPLIES: "GOD DOES CARE!"

"Likewise the Spirit also helpeth our infirmities: for we know not what we should pray for as we ought: but the Spirit itself maketh intercession for us with groanings which cannot be uttered. And he that searcheth the hearts knoweth what is the mind of the Spirit, because he maketh intercession for the saints according to the will of God." (Romans 8:26-27)

Whilst it is all good and well to talk of the Lord coming back and Christians going to Heaven, what about now? Is there any hope the

Bible gives us to cling to that has a present benefit? The answer is, "Yes!"

The Holy Spirit reminds us of a truth for every person living with bipolar to remember: God cares about everything you're going through. The Bible says that Jesus feels for us. The Holy Spirit actually prays for us when we're going through deep problems: *"the Spirit itself maketh intercession for us with groanings which cannot be uttered."(Romans 8:26)*

If you've ever been in a situation where there is so much heartache that you didn't know how to pray, that's okay. God understands the aches of your heart when you can't even verbalize it. God understands the very pain in your heart. The Holy Spirit groans out of love for us. He takes no delight in our pain and suffering. He groans over the delight of the Devil. He looks past your words and sees into your heart.

Bipolar disorder is an infirmity, a weakness, a feeble area in your life and we can have great hope because *"the Spirit also helpeth our infirmities."* The Bible teaches us that the Holy Spirit comes alongside of us and helps our infirmities. Creation groans because things aren't the way they ought to be. We groan because they aren't the way they ought to be. But here, God even feels our pain and the Holy Spirit groans for us. God is concerned about your aches and pains.

No matter what the situation, it is not hopeless because the Holy Spirit is praying for us at that moment. That's good news. God sees everything we're going through and nothing catches Him by surprise. The Bible says that when you cannot even express the hurt in your life the Holy Spirit prays for you. He looks inside your heart and sees things even you can't see, and prays them to the Heavenly Father.

I (Jenny) believe at times, when I prayed in my words, the Holy Spirit in me groaned as He knew what I really needed in that situation. As the groan was directed heavenward, where the Son is at the right hand of the Father, He rewrote it for me. He passed it to the Father and said, "Father, that is what Jenny Bakss really needs". It may not have been what I wanted, but He gives me what I need.

God looks past your words and sees into your heart. He's a good Father. Song writers Pat Barrett and Tony Brown capture the thought in their song "A Good Good Father".

> *Oh, and I've seen many searching*
> *For answers far and wide*
> *But I know we're all searching*
> *For answers only you provide*
> *'Cause You know just what we need*
> *Before we say a word*
>
> *You're a good good Father*
> *It's who You are, it's who you are, it's who you are*
> *And I'm loved by you*
> *It's who I am, it's who I am, it's who I am*

Prior to experiencing bipolar disorder, I had read John Bunyan's famous book *Pilgrim's Progress* to my young children. Then, in later years during a bipolar episode while feeling a sense of hopelessness, I recalled the time in Bunyan's allegory when the main character, Christian, fell into the slough of despond. It took Mr Hopeful to come along and pull him out. The picture of this event stuck with me and illustrated how I felt when hope vanished from my life. Thankfully, I was able to hope again and climbed out of the disgusting, slimy, mud pit in my mind.

When you are in the midst of an episode of bipolar and you're hearing the negative thoughts, just remember what hope replies - "It will cease!", "Things will change!" and "God does care!"

CHAPTER 13

GOD HAS NOT FORGOTTEN YOU

DELAY

The longest train tunnel in the world is in Switzerland and allows passengers to travel for fifty-seven kilometres (thirty-five miles) in darkness under the Swiss Alps between northern and southern Europe. In life, there are times we can feel like we are in the darkness hoping and waiting for the proverbial light at the end of the tunnel. It may be during a time of a drawn-out sickness or long-term financial problem; or maybe whilst undergoing a struggle with grief, or existing in an awful relationship that seems like a never-ending nightmare. For the person living with bipolar the tunnel goes on and on and seemingly has no end. If you have ever sparred with a mental illness, or found yourself stuck in the darkness, you can understand the psalmist David's heartfelt words and emotions.

> *"**How long** wilt thou forget me, O LORD? for ever? **how long** wilt thou hide thy face from me? **How long** shall I take counsel in my soul, having sorrow in my heart daily? **how long** shall mine enemy be exalted over me? Consider and hear me, O LORD my God: lighten mine eyes, lest I sleep the sleep of death;"* (Psalm 13:1-3)

David wrote this psalm when he was physically exhausted and emotionally depressed and felt he simply couldn't go on any farther. He experienced thoughts that the tough times would never end.

We don't know the exact circumstances of where David was when he wrote this psalm. It could have been during the eight years he was being chased by King Saul and his army, being hunted like a wild animal. It may have been the result of living through the turmoil in his own family when one of his sons raped his daughter. Perhaps it was when one of his sons, using many of his own army, revolted and tried to kill him, or when one of his sons was murdered by another. Whatever the circumstance that led to his depressed state, David felt as if it would last forever.

As parents, Jenny and I both recall the times we have taken road trips with our children and hearing the little voices from the back seat of the car asking "Are we there yet? How much longer?"

We can all at times cry out to God from the backseat of life with the same questions "How much longer, Lord?" "How much farther to go, God?" and "Lord, are we there yet?"

A family were getting together for a reunion time in New Zealand. They decided to take a walk on the beach below a rugged cliff face towards an old lighthouse. The aunt checked the tides before they set off. When halfway along the beach they noticed the tide was coming in and it seemed they would be cut off and pressed up against the cliff face. The aunt had mistakenly picked up the newspaper in the house from two weeks earlier and had the wrong tide information. The little toddlers were getting scared. The only way to safety was to climb the cliffs. The elderly started and the parents carried the children. They ended up all in various clefts of the rocks and before long the questions started to come from the lips of the panic-stricken people,

"How long before the tide goes back out?" "How long can we hang on to this cliff face?" Happily, the tide eventually turned and they were able to all get out safely.

There have been many times during Jenny's journey with bipolar that the words came ringing from our lips, "How long?" Whether it was my wife's desperate cries for relief, or my own pleas as a helpless and at times frustrated husband, we both looked for the light at the end of the tunnel.

It was during one of our searching times we found a great sense of comfort and hope from David's inspired psalm. Psalm 13 provided some much needed perspective for both of us. There were three key principles we gleaned.

PLEA TO GOD WITH DESIRE AND FEAR HIM

"How long wilt thou forget me, O LORD? for ever? how long wilt thou hide thy face from me? How long shall I take counsel in my soul, having sorrow in my heart daily? how long shall mine enemy be exalted over me?" (Psalm 13:1-2)

David here is questioning God. He is afraid, yet full of desire to seek God. In these first two verses of the psalm, David asks, *"How long?"* four times.

In the first question he is wondering if God has completely forgotten him and his plight. Having asked , *"How long?"* he immediately cries out an added question, *"For ever?"*

In David's life he had been forced to hide in caves and in the forest - not for days, weeks or months, but for years. For years, David was unable to travel freely. No wonder he asked, *"How long?"*

We all at times set time limits to our sufferings and disappointments. We feel we can hang on if it is only for a week, but when it goes on longer than expected, we reveal our demanding spirit. We conceal our demanding spirit under the guise of 'hope'. But our hope that everything will work out is really an expectation that it will happen by a certain time. When this doesn't come to pass we get discouraged and frustrated. Praying seems useless, as though God cannot hear us. It is a silence that is deafening. Hope of coming out of the depressive episode seems nowhere to be found.

In the early years of our journey with bipolar we thought it was only a temporary thing and Jenny would 'snap out of it'. As time dragged on and Jenny didn't improve or show any signs of change - in fact she got worse - I felt God had forgotten us and wasn't hearing our prayers. My prayers began to change from "God we trust you" to "God you've got to do something soon".

We see this attitude in the life of the Old Testament person of Job. After the terrible tragedies in his life in losing his wealth then his children, Job confessed. *"...Naked came I out of my mother's womb, and naked shall I return thither: the LORD gave, and the LORD hath taken away; blessed be the name of the LORD. In all this Job sinned not, nor charged God foolishly." (Job 1:21-22)*

Then he also lost his health and finally his wife cracked under the intense emotional pressure and suggested he curse God and die. Job replied to his wife's anguish, *"Thou speakest as one of the foolish women speaketh. What? shall we receive good at the hand of God,* and shall we not receive evil? In all this did not Job sin with his lips." (Job 2:10)

As time drew on and nothing changed in Job's circumstances he began to change his tune. *"Oh that I might have my request; and that God would grant me the thing that I long for!" (Job 6:8)* He then started to demand to speak to God. *"Surely I would speak to the Almighty, and I desire to reason with God." (Job 13:3)* But he thought God was not listening. *"Behold, I cry out of wrong, but I am not heard: I cry aloud, but there is no judgment." (Job 19:7)* Finally the time-delay exposed his demanding spirit. *"Even to day is my complaint bitter: my stroke is heavier than my groaning. Oh that I knew where I might find him! that I might come even to his seat! I would order my cause before him, and fill my mouth with arguments." (Job 23:2-4)*

It is in these moments where our grumbling turns into murmuring against God. We can start to think, "How long am I going to pray and go to church and not seem like I'm getting anything from you?" "How long am I going to have to wrestle with my thoughts of 'What if' and 'If only'?" When there seems to be a delay, we may go through the same emotions as David.

We feel Forgotten - *"How long wilt thou forget me, O LORD? for ever?"* v.1a

We may come to the point where we think God has forgotten us. Perhaps our problems aren't important to Him. Everyone has a point somewhere in the geography of their souls marking the limits of their faith. It is at this point that faith begins to unravel and we can begin to give up on God, thinking that God has given up on us. It is in these moments we must remember that God will never forget us. Even though a mother could possibly forget her own child, our God will never forget His children. God has not forgotten you! *"Can a woman forget her sucking child, that she should not have compassion on the son of her womb? yea, they may forget, yet will I not forget thee."* (Isaiah 49:15)

We feel Forsaken – *"how long wilt thou hide thy face from me?" v.1b*

David felt God has purposely turned away from him and could not be bothered by his problems. Yet, despite what we may feel, we know that God has said, *"...I will never leave thee, nor forsake thee."* (Hebrews 13:5)

We feel Frustrated – *"How long shall I take counsel in my soul, having sorrow in my heart daily? how long shall mine enemy be exalted over me?" v.2*

Those suffering from a bipolar episode can feel as David felt - that everyday was another day of the same 'daily' heartache. He felt he had no one to talk to but himself. He was frustrated to think that his enemies were rejoicing in his plight. When I (Jenny) am in a low state for a prolonged period there is a level of frustration in feeling that nobody understands what I am going through. The inner conversations with myself can switch from negative and self-condemning to being judgemental and angry at others. I have found when my emotions take over, it is always hard to get back on to a level course. It is during these moments the fear of God motivates me to make my plea to God with desire for change knowing that He has not forgotten or forsaken me.

PRAY TO GOD FOR DIRECTION TO FOLLOW HIM

"Consider and hear me, O LORD my God: lighten mine eyes, lest I sleep the sleep of death; Lest mine enemy say, I have prevailed against him; and those that trouble me rejoice when I am moved." (Psalm 13:3-4)

Like David in this psalm, we found prayer was like a pressure relief valve in our lives. Whilst the bipolar was still present, when we prayed it became medicine to the soul to know that our heavenly Father was listening to our heart cry.

Notice the little word *"lest"* in David's prayer. It is like he is saying, "Unless you help, I'm done for, Lord. I am going to die under this burden if You don't help me." In another of David's psalms he echoes a similar sentiment, *"I had fainted, unless I had believed to see the goodness of the LORD in the land of the living." (Psalm 27:13)*

Have you ever felt you were under such a heavy load that you thought if it was not lifted, it would destroy you? We have, during many of the prolonged depressive episodes. Some depression sufferers have called these times 'the dark night of the soul.' As hard as the trials were, we have discovered the episodes were often secondary, and that God used them to bring about spiritual strength. It was in these dark hours that we were both brought to a place of dependence upon God.

I (Robert) clearly recall a time during a depressive episode when Jenny had gone to stay with her parents for some respite and quiet rest. She was still not well and some dear friends of ours offered to drive her the eight hour journey back home. Unbeknown to me, while travelling home they encountered a severe storm which prohibited them from continuing the journey. They were forced to pull over for the night and rest in the friends' caravan they were towing until the storm passed. There were no mobile phones in those days and hence I received no phone call to alert me to what had happened. Several hours had passed after the original estimated arrival time and I began to become very concerned. I remember telephoning Police stations to find out if an accident had been reported. In the midst of the stress and worry, I realised I hadn't called on the one person who can calm the troubled soul – God. I immediately spent time in prayer and poured out my concerns to the Lord. A peace flooded my heart and soul and I was able to rest knowing that all was in the Father's hands. Within an hour I received a phone call from one of the friends who explained their delay.

We've often noticed how God steers us into an emotional cul-de-sac and it seems like He corrals us into a corner until we realise we have nowhere else to turn, but to Him!

It is essential in our dark times that we maintain a right view of God. When David prayed *"O LORD my God"* he was adjusting his focus from his trouble on to the One who could help him in his trouble.

It is in these moments of darkness we can pray for three things, as David did:

- Look on me God – *"**consider** me Lord"*

- Listen to me God – *"Lord, please, **hear** me"*

- Lead me God – *"**lighten** mine eyes Lord, put some light back into my path and way"*

When we feel forgotten and delays happen or expectations fail, our response will reflect our view of the will of God. We must remember that if our theology is wrong, our philosophy on life will be wrong. If our view of God is that He is a distant and at times absent God, we will feel forgotten and forsaken. However, if our view is that *"God is our refuge and strength, a very present help in trouble." (Psalm 46:1)*, then we believe that God fully knows what He is doing.

We must get to the place where we take our burdens to the Lord and allow them to become prayers. God comes to our aid. He is waiting for this pressing issue, this trouble, to become a prayer. He is waiting for us to cry out to Him, seeking Him for help.

As a couple, we have learnt to never accept our problems as the end of it all, but to see them as tools in the hand of God to bring us closer to Him. During the lows of bipolar, I (Jenny) often can't think very clearly to make sound decisions and, like David in this psalm, I pray to the Lord believing He will answer my prayers and show me the path I should follow. I need someone to tell me what to do and that someone is God.

Believing God can direct our path enables us to do the final thing seen in this psalm.

PRAISE GOD FOR DELIVERANCE THROUGH FAITH IN HIM

"But I have trusted in thy mercy; my heart shall rejoice in thy salvation. I will sing unto the LORD, because he hath dealt bountifully with me." (Psalm 13:5-6)

The prayer no longer dwells on how long David has suffered, but rather shifts to him trusting in God's unfailing love. There's nothing like dwelling on where God has brought you from, to be appreciative of where you are right now. When David began praising the Lord in this psalm, he emphasised both the mercy of God and the goodness of God. It is one thing to have God deal with you; it is another thing to have God deal bountifully with you. David recalled how God had been with him in the past and recognised by faith He would not leave Him now.

God is concerned with ALL that concerns us and we are encouraged to give all our cares and worries to the Lord because He cares for us. *"Casting all your care upon him; for he careth for you." (1 Peter 5:7)* To know that God is as concerned with my bipolar disorder as I am, gave me comfort.

The apostle John gives us the shortest verse in the Bible that may be the most profound of all: *"Jesus wept" (John 11:35)*. While Jesus Himself was not depressed, He still wept with Mary and Martha when they were grieving after Lazarus died. He ministered to many other people who were depressed, like the woman with the blood disorder, the paralytic at the Sheep Gate pool and the self-mutilator who lived in the tombs. Jesus knows and cares about people living with depression. *"The LORD is nigh unto them that are of a broken heart; and saveth such as be of a contrite spirit." (Psalm 34:18)*

Too many people with bipolar disorder feel as if God has forsaken them in their sickness, but that just isn't true. He is still with them, even through their disorder. *"(For the LORD thy God is a merciful God;) he will not forsake thee..." (Deuteronomy 4:31)*

I (Jenny) recently heard a song called "I will follow you" that encapsulates this thought in the lyrics:

> *I believe everything that You say You are*
> *I believe that I have seen Your unchanging heart*
> *In the good things and in the hardest part*
> *I believe and I will follow You*[26]

It is no longer, "God has forgotten me," but rather, "God is very near". He's only a prayer away. I have come to know that God is right here with me even in the bipolar episodes that seem to never end. Each time I'm feeling depressed and downcast I simply need to move from *"How long?"* to *"He hath dealt bountifully with me."*

---

26 "I will follow" by Vertical Church Band. https://www.youtube.com/watch?v=Xh3ZK7JecK0

The story is told of a Sunday Bible class that had been asked the question, "In your time of discouragement, what is your favourite scripture?" A young man said, *"The LORD is my shepherd; I shall not want." (Psalm 23:1)* A middle aged woman said, *"God is our refuge and strength, a very present help in trouble." (Psalm 46:1)* Another woman said, *"These things I have spoken unto you, that in me ye might have peace. In the world ye shall have tribulation: but be of good cheer; I have overcome the world." (John 16:33)* Then John, an eighty-year-old man said, "It's a phase in a verse that's my favourite, *'and it came to pass'* and it occurs 396 times in the King James Bible." The class started to laugh a little, thinking that old John's lack of memory was getting the best of him. When the snickering stopped, he said. "At thirty, I lost my job with six hungry mouths and a wife to feed. I didn't know how I would make it. At forty, my eldest son was killed overseas in the war. It knocked me down. At fifty, my house burned to the ground. Nothing was saved out of the house. At sixty, my wife of forty years got cancer. It slowly ate away at her. We cried together many a night on our knees in prayer. At sixty-five, she died. I still miss her today. The agony I went through in each of these situations was unbelievable. I wondered where God was. But each time I looked in the Bible I saw one of those 396 verses that said, *"and it came to pass."* I felt that God was telling me my pain and my circumstances were also going to pass, and that God would get me through it."

There's something about knowing the love of God and understanding the promise of Jesus to never leave nor forsake us, that makes us want to sing of God's goodness in our lives.

CHAPTER 14

MAKING SOME SENSE OF SUFFERING

DESIGN

Mental illness is not all bad. In fact I (Jenny) have found it has many benefits. I'm not unhappy with my life and in many ways I value what bipolar has made possible for me. However, I wasn't always able to say those words, until I came to the understanding that God has a purpose and plan even in our suffering.

One day while reading through the gospel of John, I came across a passage of scripture that made me wonder if there was a grander design for my sickness.

> "Now a certain man was sick, named Lazarus, of Bethany, the town of Mary and her sister Martha. (It was that Mary which anointed the Lord with ointment, and wiped his feet with her hair, whose brother Lazarus was sick.) Therefore his sisters sent unto him, saying, Lord, behold, he whom thou lovest is sick. When Jesus heard that, he said, This sickness is not unto death, but for the glory of God, that the Son of God might be glorified thereby." (John 11:1-4)

It was the words of Jesus giving purpose to the sickness of Lazarus that made me ask, "Could it be that my sickness is *for the glory of*

God? Could there be a divine purpose to having bipolar? Could my bipolar be a gift in disguise? Can I make some sense of my suffering?"

These and many other questions began to flood my mind. I eventually came to accept the way God, the great potter, had made me His special vessel for His glory.

We all know that pain and suffering will be a part of life. Living with bipolar certainly has its share of trouble. Trouble is an inescapable reality in this fallen, evil world. From someone who knew a little bit about trouble and suffering, Job in the Old Testament reminds us all, *"Man that is born of a woman is of few days, and full of trouble." (Job 14:1)* Jeremiah, the weeping prophet, lamented, *"Wherefore came I forth out of the womb to see labour and sorrow, that my days should be consumed with shame?" (Jeremiah 20:18)*

The question remains, "How do we make some sense of suffering?"

To begin answering this question, let's consider an amazing illustration from God's creation. Zoologist and author, Gary Richmond, tells about the birth of a giraffe: The first thing to emerge are the baby giraffe's front hooves and head. A few minutes later the plucky newborn calf is hurled forth, falls ten feet and lands on its back. Within seconds, he rolls to an upright position with his legs tucked under his body. From this position he considers the world for the first time and shakes off the last vestiges of the birthing fluid from his eyes and ears. The mother giraffe lowers her head long enough to take a quick look. Then she positions herself directly over her calf. She waits for about a minute and then she does the most unreasonable thing. She swings her long, pendulous leg outward and kicks her baby, so that it is sent sprawling head over heels. When it doesn't get up, the violent process is repeated over and over again. The struggle to rise is momentous. As the baby calf grows tired, the mother kicks it again to stimulate its efforts. Finally, the calf stands for the first time on its wobbly legs. Then the mother giraffe does the most remarkable thing. She kicks it off its feet again. [27]

Maybe you can somehow relate to the calf. It's not that you were kicked over and over again by your mother when you were born, but we can relate to the calf when it comes to the problems, difficulties and trials that hit us in life. Some problems are sometimes so big that they send us sprawling head over heels.

Problems or discouragements are no respecter of persons, whether you are successful or not, rich or poor, healthy or ill, etc, you will experience them.

The apostle Paul wrote to the Corinthians recounting his personal experiences and teaches us three principles we can learn from our suffering.

RECOGNISE THE WAYS COMFORT IS EXPERIENCED FROM GOD

"Blessed be God, even the Father of our Lord Jesus Christ, the Father of mercies, and the God of all comfort; Who comforteth us in all our tribulation,..." (2 Corinthians 1:3-4a)

Since so much of his letter focussed on pain, suffering and heartache, it's not surprising that Paul began by explaining some of the reasons we experience trials. The word 'comfort' almost leaps off the page. It is key to Paul's explanation.

---

27 "A View from the Zoo" Gary Richmond, W Pub Group (September 1987)

What do we mean by comfort? What's our idea of comfort?

Sometimes we have an idea that comfort is taking away the problem or trouble that we are experiencing, somewhat like dental treatment can take away the pain of a toothache. This is not God's idea of comfort. God's comfort describes conquering rather than convenience. We cry out "Take it away God!" to which He replies *"My grace is sufficient for thee: for my strength is made perfect in weakness." (2 Corinthians 12:9)*

The word 'comfort' or 'consolation' is used ten times in the first chapter of this letter to the Corinthians and means "to call to one's side." Comfort is given by someone called alongside to help - like a nurse called to a patient's bedside.

Comfort does not remove our sufferings or our difficulties, but rather it brings us the strength, encouragement and hope to deal with them. When tragedy strikes, collapsing our life like a house of cards, comfort is what we need most. We need someone to come alongside and put an arm around us, to be there, to listen and to help. We need the Comforter, the Father of mercies and the God of all comfort and He promises us His presence.

Many seek comfort in all the wrong people and places, often creating even more problems and suffering. The vulnerability of having bipolar makes a person susceptible to wrong choices as a source of comfort. Sadly, some times the bipolar sufferer becomes the victim of predatory behaviour that extends a false hope of comfort.

Many times in a depressed episode of bipolar, people will look to sleep as their elixir of comfort only to find themselves waking still plagued with dark thoughts. They can possibly relate to the words of Job in his quest for comfort. *"When I say, My bed shall comfort me, my couch shall ease my complaint; Then thou scarest me with dreams,* and terrifiest me through visions: So that my soul chooseth strangling, and death rather than my life. I loathe it; I would not live alway: let me alone; for my days are vanity."(Job 7:13-16) In my darkest times during the early onset of bipolar disorder I (Jenny) would occasionally hear voices in my head and my mind would begin to think of self-harm and sometimes evil thoughts.

I (Robert) remember a time coming into our bedroom one evening and finding Jenny sitting cross-legged on the bed with her back up against the head board. Her eyes told the story. I could tell she was not in a clear frame of mind and her thoughts were morbid. Her countenance was one of anger, which was not the normal Jenny I knew. When Jenny got into such a state, I could just see it in her eyes. It made me think of what Jesus said, *"The light of the body is the eye: if therefore thine eye be single, thy whole body shall be full of light. But if thine eye be evil, thy whole body shall be full of darkness. If therefore the light that is in thee be darkness, how great is that darkness!"* (Matthew 6:22-23)

I (Jenny) felt numbness. I had nothing to give. I couldn't stand for Robert or the children to come near me or touch me because I felt I had nothing to give back. I am thankful to say God rescued me out from this deep dark pit. Praise His name!

True comfort comes from God Whom the apostle Paul calls the *"God of all comfort"*. Comfort is just one of His many mercies. He can provide ALL comfort to which there is no limitation. As we look to the Word of God we can glean at least seven key sources that God uses to provide comfort to the sufferer.

Scriptures are a source of comfort - *"For whatsoever things were written aforetime were written for our learning, that we through patience and comfort of the scriptures might have hope."* (Romans 15:4)

Throughout the journey with bipolar, I (Jenny) have gained great comfort from many verses of scripture which have each become special to me. These verses deal primarily with the mind and fear. Some of the verses include:

> "For God hath not given us the spirit of fear; but of power, and of love, and of a sound mind." (2 Timothy 1:7)

> "And be renewed in the spirit of your mind;" (Ephesians 4:23)

> "Casting down imaginations, and every high thing that exalteth itself against the knowledge of God, and bringing into captivity every thought to the obedience of Christ;" (2 Corinthians 10:5)

> "What time I am afraid, I will trust in thee." (Psalm 56:3)

> "Finally, brethren, whatsoever things are true, whatsoever things are honest, whatsoever things are just, whatsoever things are pure, whatsoever things are lovely, whatsoever things are of good report; if there be any virtue, and if there be any praise, think on these things." (Philippians 4:8)

Songs are a source of comfort – "But none saith, Where is God my maker, who giveth songs in the night;" (Job 35:10)

Music has always been a great comfort to me. Sitting down and listening to psalms, hymns and spiritual songs calms my thoughts. I feel at times like Elisha in the Old Testament when he was refreshed by music. "But now bring me a minstrel. And it came to pass, when the minstrel played, that the hand of the LORD came upon him." (2 Kings 3:15)

A song that provided tremendous measure of comfort during one particular bad episode of bipolar depression is called "He knows my name" written by Tommy Walker.

I don't know what tomorrow will bring, I can't tell you what's in store
I don't know a lot of things, I don't have all the answers
To the questions of my life, But I know in Whom I have believed

And he knows my name
Every step that I take
Every move that I make
Every tear that I cry
He knows my name
When I'm overwhelmed by the pain
And can't see the light of day
I know I'll be just fine
'Cause he knows my name

Staff of God is a source of comfort - *"Yea, though I walk through the valley of the shadow of death, I will fear no evil: for thou art with me; thy rod and thy staff they comfort me." (Psalm 23:4)*

The shepherd's staff is a source of comfort for the sheep because the sheep know the shepherd will use the staff to protect, guide and deliver them. So too, God's hand of protection, guidance and deliverance through the people He brings into your life and through the providential moments of life, each bring comfort.

Sustenance (food) is a source of comfort - *"And it came to pass on the fourth day, when they arose early in the morning, that he rose up to depart: and the damsel's father said unto his son in law, Comfort thine heart with a morsel of bread, and afterward go your way." (Judges 19:5)*

We often hear about emotional eating of 'comfort food' in a negative connotation. However, there are times when living with bipolar that good nutritious food is a much needed source of comfort physically. When Jenny was in a prolonged low period of depression, her appetite went from her and she lost nearly half her body weight over a period of six months. It was during this time that I (Robert) would ensure she would continue to eat wholesome meals which slowly nourished her back to physical strength.

Saints of God are a source of comfort – *"Nevertheless God, that comforteth those that are cast down, comforted us by the coming of Titus;" (2 Corinthians 7:6)*

Until you hit rock bottom and lie in a 'slough of despond', you never truly appreciate the great comfort that God's people can bring to your life. To know people are praying for your well-being and care enough to contact you in your high and low episodes is a constant supply of comfort. I (Jenny) have been blessed with some precious Christian women friends who embody the proverb: *"A friend loveth at all times, and a brother is born for adversity." (Proverbs 17:17)* Besides my family, some of my dear friends who have always been there for me from the onset of my illness include, Leanne Gray, Coral Ruff and Kay Hooper. These ladies have been a tower of strength to me helping with practical tasks, praying and counselling with me.

Spouses are a source of comfort – *"And Isaac brought her into his mother Sarah's tent, and took Rebekah, and she became his wife; and he loved her: and Isaac was comforted after his mother's death." (Genesis 24:67)*

To know you have a spouse who seeks to understand your illness is a blessing of comfort that no one else can provide. Robert has always stood with me, behind me and beside me in every episode of bipolar.

His patience during the trying times comforted my heart and soul when it seemed everything was hopeless.

Spirit of God is a the source of comfort - *"And I will pray the Father, and he shall give you another Comforter, that he may abide with you for ever;" (John 14:16)*

A relationship with the Holy Spirit of God is imperative for any sufferer, for it is the function of the Holy Spirit who indwells the believer to come alongside and speak peace to your heart and mind. He gives grace and peace that is a supernatural work in your life. *"And the peace of God, which passeth all understanding, shall keep your hearts and minds through Christ Jesus." (Philippians 4:7)*

REALISE THE COMFORT IS FOR YOU TO EXTEND TO OTHERS

Have you ever known people who despite tragedy were able to offer comfort to others? On the other hand, some people are devastated by personal hardships and find no peace, no consolation. They certainly are in no position to help others. What is the difference? Where do those who are able to comfort others while enduring their tragedy receive the strength to help others? The apostle Paul was one individual who had learned the secret and he passed it along to us in his second letter to the Corinthians. Continuing on after referring to the God of all comfort, Paul writes:

> *"Who comforteth us in all our tribulation, **that we may be able to comfort them** which are in any trouble, by the comfort wherewith we ourselves are comforted of God. For as the sufferings of Christ abound in us, so our consolation also*

*aboundeth by Christ. And whether we be afflicted, **it is for your consolation** and salvation, which is effectual in the enduring of the same sufferings which we also suffer: or whether we be comforted, **it is for your consolation** and salvation. And our hope of you is stedfast, knowing, that as ye are partakers of the sufferings, so shall ye be also of the consolation." (2 Corinthians 1:4b-7)*

The principle of these verses is simply stated: Don't waste your pain.

This comfort that we receive from God is not simply for our personal enjoyment. It is given to us that we might be able to help others. "*… that we may be able to comfort them which are in any trouble, by the comfort wherewith we ourselves are comforted of God.*" This is also one of the reasons God allows us to go through certain trials in life. When you experience problems and difficulties in life, remember that God can use you to extend His comfort to others going through the same difficulty. Great encouragers are those who have experienced great tribulations.

Sir Edmund Hillary and his Nepalese guide, Tenzing Norgay, were the first people to make the historic climb of Mount Everest in 1953. Coming down from the mountain peak, Sir Edmund suddenly lost his footing. Tenzing held the line taut and kept them both from falling by digging his axe into the ice. Later Tenzing refused any special credit for saving Sir Edmund Hillary's life; he considered it a routine part of the job. As he put it, "Mountain climbers always help each other."[28]

We are to help one another and comfort one another by sharing our experiences. We don't just give others empathy and sympathy but we

---

28 Words of Power: 365 Inspirational Messages, Jeanne Alcott, Day 13. WestBow Press, 2014

are to give them HOPE. We comfort others by referring them to the sources and ways that God has comforted us. We cannot lead others where we have not been ourselves.

I (Jenny) have found it gives comfort to other bipolar sufferers to let them know that it is okay to be a Christian and have a mental illness. One reason God allows suffering is so we might have a deep well of experiences from which to draw compassion and counsel for others. I'm thankful my bipolar has created a compassion for others who suffer from depression and other mental health issues. God has shown me His love and comfort and I want to pass this on to others.

I've been fortunate to be part of a church community that has supported me and helped me grow spiritually through my illness. During one very trying episode, a dear lady in the church organised for different people to make an evening meal to be delivered to our home, for an entire month. Their kindness is recorded in heaven forever. With the Christ-like love they have shown me, I have come to understand how great God's love is. In turn, I now help others through one-on-one support. The language of suffering I've learned helps me connect with people afflicted with similar troubles. I am able to understand them in a way many others could not.

In 1998, the late Robin Williams starred in a movie call "Patch Adams" which was based on the true life story of Dr Hunter "Patch" Adams. Patch was admitted to a psychiatric hospital after failed suicide attempts. While Patch was a patient, he discovered his ability to connect with people through humour. He learned to understand his severely disturbed roommate, to see the person behind the illness, and helped him through his problems. Not only did this delight Patch; it made him a well man. Patch eagerly told his doctor he was well and needed to leave the hospital. "I connected to another human being", he said. "I want to do more of that. I want to learn about people. I want to help them with their troubles. I want to really listen to people." Connecting with other people gave Patch joy.

It gives me great joy to be able to help others and connect to others *"by the comfort wherewith we ourselves are comforted of God."* When God places you in the lives of others who are struggling with a similar pain and suffering, suddenly you realise your suffering makes some sense. Walking with people through some of their toughest times is rewarding and a privilege. Bipolar disorder will always be with me and I suffer many high and low moods. But I don't feel I'm a victim of the disorder. God has helped me find a way to make my illness work for me instead of against me.

God has a design and plan for each of us. Even though I have a severe illness, God has work for me to do. For all those who also suffer with a mental illness and gain comfort from God, be encouraged that you can use what God has given you, even the bad and be turned into something good. God said to the suffering prophet Jeremiah, *"For I know the thoughts that I think toward you, saith the LORD, thoughts of peace, and not of evil, to give you an expected end."* (Jeremiah 29:11).

Suffering prepares us to comfort others. Someone who has suffered the shattering effects of a divorce is the best person to comfort a divorcee. The parent who has lost a child can best comfort another grieving parent. The businessman who once was bankrupt can best comfort another person in the throes of financial disaster.

I recognised that suffering will always be a part of my life, yet I am rich on so many fronts. Like many people who suffer with bipolar, I am a very creative person. I love my crafts, knitting, sewing, cooking, card-making, gardening and taking photos using my imagination. During my time in hospital, I have been able to teach others the

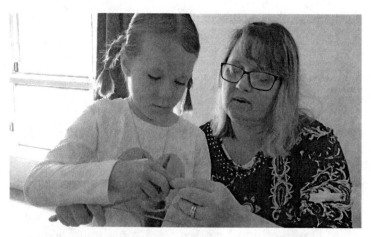

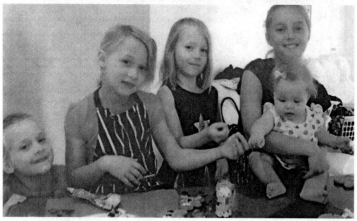

Fun times knitting and cooking with Grandma

almost lost art of knitting. I constantly look for ways to use my creative bent to encourage other bipolar sufferers.

I remember a time when my beloved doctor, Dr Sandy Prasad, said to me, "Jenny when you are having a low episode God will help you through it, and when you are feeling great, just enjoy the moments and live it up, girl!" The difficult dark days have helped me appreciate the good bright days and I make the most of them.

The next time suffering shows up in your life, try implementing these three suggestions:

- Instead of focusing only on yourself, think of how you can help others later. This will sound a note of hope.

- Rather than fighting, surrender; rather than resisting, release. This will produce a note of faith.

- Although getting even seems to come more naturally, try giving thanks. This will bring a note of peace. Count your many blessings and write them down.

RELY ON GOD ALONE AND EXALT HIM WHILST LIVING WITH BIPOLAR

*"For we would not, brethren, have you ignorant of our trouble which came to us in Asia, that we were pressed out of measure, above strength, insomuch that we despaired even of life: But we had the sentence of death in ourselves, **that we should not trust in ourselves, but in God** which raiseth the dead: Who delivered us from so great a death, and doth deliver: in whom we trust that he will yet deliver us; Ye also helping together by prayer for us, that for the gift bestowed upon us by the means of many persons thanks may be given by many on our behalf." (2 Corinthians 1:8)*

Paul bared his heart here and shared with the believers the troubles he endured in Asia. Whatever these troubles were, they were sufficient to crush Paul and cause him to pass sentence on his life. He despaired even of life itself. How comforting to know that even the great saints of God are still made of clay. He wrote this, not to win their sympathy, but to teach them the lesson he learned – trust God alone.

The trials have really created a greater dependence on God. Knowing that He has brought us both through every low and high episode strengthens our faith in God.

Our struggles and growth with bipolar have been ongoing, but just like the apostle Paul learned the lesson God had for him, we too do not trust in ourselves, but in God alone. Suffering keeps us from trusting in ourselves. Intense suffering is designed to remind us of our utter helplessness, for it is when we are most helpless that we are most dependent. Jenny's life scripture verses are, *"Trust in the LORD with all thine heart; and lean not unto thine own understanding. In all thy ways acknowledge him, and he shall direct thy paths." (Proverbs 3:5-6)*

I (Robert) know that Jenny could have used her illness as reason to give up and resign herself to a life of misery without any purpose to the pain. Yet she is my number one hero, because a hero is someone who has succeeded while struggling with the same problems others have used as excuses for failure.

I (Jenny) don't know why God allowed me to have bipolar disorder. I prayed for healing many times in the beginning. I don't believe that Jesus' healing powers were limited to His three years of ministry on earth. God is well able to heal today if He chooses to do so. Our eldest son Ben, at the age of twelve was stricken with Bell's palsy. Our doctor explained that the stroke-like symptoms down the left side of his face could be permanent. We had our church family and many others pray for his healing. Within two weeks the virus that caused the illness disappeared. Then why hasn't the Lord seen fit to heal me of bipolar? I'm confident now that He has a greater design and my bipolar will be a "thorn in the flesh" for His glory. With this in mind I am resolved to say, like Paul, *"Most gladly therefore will I rather glory in my infirmities, that the power of Christ may rest upon me." (2 Corinthians 12:9b)*

The Bible also says that *"And we know that all things work together for good to them that love God, to them who are the called according to his purpose." (Romans 8:28)* "All things" includes even my bipolar disorder.

I know that my bipolar has definitely made me a stronger person, for what I have had to go through and what I have had to fight.

Going back to the giraffe story from earlier, the mother giraffe kicks her calf off its feet again. Why? She wants it to remember how it got up. In the world, a baby giraffe must be able to get up as quickly as possible in order to stay with the herd, where there is safety. Lions, hyenas, leopards and wild hunting dogs all enjoy eating young giraffes and hunt them down. The mother needed to teach her calf to get up quickly and keep within the safety of the herd.

There have been many times when it seemed that both Robert and I had just stood up after a trial, only to be knocked down again by the next. We now know it was our loving God helping us to remember how it was that we got up, urging us always to walk with him, in His shadow, under His care.

Our daughter-in-law, Alice, once wrote to me and said:

> *"Hey! I just wanted to say – in case you didn't know - that even with your bipolar moments that we laugh about and you can't remember, you are unbelievably precious to both Ben and myself and I have learnt so much about graciousness and gentleness from you since I had the honour of becoming one of your daughters. I know how hard it is being you (it rivals how hard it is being me) especially on those really hard low days. But once you overcome you never complain, you just carry on. In my books this makes you one of the strongest women I know. You did an awesome job raising my husband to be the man he is today. I love you (and dad) to absolute pieces. xxx"*

CHAPTER 15

HOW TO BEAT THE BLUES

DEPRESSION

We all have bad days and for some of us those bad days have stretched into bad weeks, months or even years. We find ourselves talking like Eeyore and saying things like, "Whatever can go wrong will go wrong."

We have a pessimistic, browbeaten, downcast view of life. We suddenly find that we can't sleep, we've lost (or gained) weight and some days we just don't want to get out of bed. If you can relate to what we are talking about, then you might just be depressed.

Some bristle when we say that. There's a part of man that simply does not want to, or is not willing to, admit to having depression. Many Christians deny that it's possible for a believer and some even look on depression as a sin. Over the course of my ministry experience as a pastor, I (Robert) have heard people say something like, "I'm a Christian and Christians can't be depressed." Christians feel bad when we have depression and feel obligated to hide it. We don't want God to look bad. When asked, "How are you?" the depressed Christian puts on the mask and gives a fake cheerful reply "Oh, I'm blessed", yet they walk away sad.

You might be surprised to know that God's people have a long and distinguished history of going through times of deep depression. Depression is no respecter of persons. It invades the lives of all people, no matter what their station in life is.

Astronaut Buzz (Edwin Eugene) Aldrin Jr., was a Lunar Module Pilot on Apollo 11 and was one of the first two humans to land on the moon. Neil Armstrong was first to set foot on the moon and Buzz was second. He returned to earth and found that he couldn't cope with the life to which he returned and went into bouts of serious depression. He later went onto talk shows to share his experience.

One of the 'greats' of human history, the British bulldog, Sir Winston Churchill suffered terribly from depression. He said it followed him like 'a black dog.'

The 16th President of the United States of America, Abraham Lincoln, whose "House divided against itself", speech helped to win him the presidency, knew awful divisive doubt and depression in his own life.

Charles Haddon Spurgeon, one of the greatest preachers of all time, who was known for his sparkling wit and quick humour, nevertheless had a lifetime battle with depression which was caused by gout, the disease which led to his death at the age of 58. He shocked his listeners when he said this in a sermon: "I am the subject of depressions of spirit so fearful that I hope none of you ever get to such extremes of wretchedness as I go through."

Both unipolar and bipolar depression are complicated, multifaceted mental health conditions. Unipolar depression is a set of symptoms someone with a major depressive episode is experiencing, which suggests a diagnosis of major depressive disorder. Conversely, someone with bipolar depression is likely experiencing both a major depressive episode and a manic episode, suggesting a diagnosis of bipolar disorder.

Being depressed is not inherently sinful and depression is not always caused by sin, nor does it indicate a lack of faith. When depression strikes, the sufferer needs to make discovering the cause and treatment of the depression a priority.

This is what we know about depression in general...

Depression is an old problem. It's not just common to the fast-paced society in which we live. From the very beginning, people have been depressed. Hippocrates, the ancient physician, because of depression being so common in his day, wrote a treatise on the melancholy spirit. The old testament prophet Elijah got depressed and we read one of his private moments. He was wanting to die and cried out to God; *"But he himself went a day's journey into the wilderness, and came and sat down under a juniper tree: and **he requested for himself that he might die**; and said, **It is enough**; now, O LORD, **take away my life**; for I am not better than my fathers." (1 Kings 19:4)* He was fully immersed in depression. This is where you say, "I can't deal with this". You're afraid to answer the phone, afraid to open another envelope. You don't want to go to work and don't know what else you are going to face. You come to the point in life where you say *"It is enough".* Depression can be one of Satan's tools to take Christians out of the work of the Lord and can affect our view of God and sap our joy.

Depression is an ordinary problem. It is a universal problem. It is no respecter of persons, places, cultures, or times. Millions of people, including Christians, suffer from depression every day. It's not something that just happens in pressure-packed lives. The following are some statistics on Depression in Australia.[29]

---

29 National Survey of Mental Health and Wellbeing, Australian Bureau of Statistics

- Depression and anxiety are the most prevalent mental disorders experienced by Australians. Depression alone is predicted to be one of the world's largest health problems by 2020.

- Around one million Australian adults and 100,000 young people live with depression each year.

- On average, one in five people will experience depression in their lives; one in four females and one in six males.

- Among young Australians aged 12-25 years, depression is the most common mental health problem.

- Around one-in-ten young Australians will experience an anxiety disorder in any given 12- month period.

- At least one third of young people have had an episode of mental illness by the age of 25 years.

- Mental disorders and suicide account for 14.2% of Australia's total health burden, which equates to 374,541 years of healthy life lost.

- Estimates suggest that up to 75% of people presenting with alcohol and drug problems also have additional mental health problems.

- Reports indicate that up to 85% of homeless people have a mental illness.[30]

Depression is an overall problem. It doesn't just come to the lower classes of people, or people who have lost their jobs or are poor. As we read through God's word, we find that many of the great men in the Bible were not immune to depression. John the Baptist

---

30 https://mhaustralia.org/sites/default/files/imported/component/rsfiles/factsheets/ statistics_on_mental_health.pdf

understandably got depressed when he lay in his cell wondering what the Messiah was doing. Jeremiah wept copiously over the destruction of Jerusalem and when his own circumstances went from bad to worse. Job scratched himself with a broken piece of pottery and listened to his depressing friends give their advice. Elijah fell into a dark hole of depression after his victory on Mount Carmel.

What is depression? It can be defined by feelings of dejection, apathy, inertia, difficulty in gaining energy or excitement, fatigue, pessimism, fear, attitudes of worthlessness, loss of interest, inability to experience pleasure and a loss of self-esteem. It is often accompanied by a feeling of helplessness, overwhelmed by circumstances, withdrawal and isolation. Left unchecked, this sadness can turn to hostility and hopelessness.

As a pastor, I (Robert) have met people who were struggling with depression who thought they were merely sad and discouraged. On the other hand, I've also counselled with some people who were extremely sad and worried they might be depressed. The reason for the confusion is because we associate depression with its primary symptom of pervasive sadness which can lead to both depression or to general discouragement.

Sadness is a *normal* human emotion. We've all experienced it and we all will again. Sadness is usually triggered by a difficult, hurtful, challenging, or disappointing event, experience, trauma or situation. In other words, we tend to feel sad about *something*. This also means that when that something changes, when our emotional hurt fades, when we've adjusted or gotten over the loss or disappointment, our sadness leaves.

Depression is an *abnormal* emotional state, a mental illness that affects our thinking, emotions, perceptions, and behaviours in pervasive and chronic ways. When we're depressed we feel sad about *everything*. Depression can be the result of circumstances triggering a major depressive episode but it does not necessarily require a difficult event or situation, a loss, or a change of circumstance as a trigger. In fact, it often occurs in the absence of any such triggers.

Depression is often associated with sadness, but it goes much further. Depression is more intense, it lasts longer and, most telling, it interferes with our ability to function. Depression is associated with deep trouble and feeling dysfunctional whilst discouragement is short term and not as debilitating. We all have times of sadness, but depression gets in the way of normal life activities.

Continual discouragement may lead a person into a state of depression. Depression is a specific alteration of a person's mood in a downward direction. People suffering from depression are often prone to extreme tiredness, overeating or sudden weight loss, worry, loss of sex drive, uncontrolled or inappropriate episodes of crying and withdrawal from social activities, friends and family.

Depression is a silent killer. You wake up in the morning and can't get away from it. You are at lunch with your friends and it's constantly nagging you inside. You are at your child's sports game and you have this constant feeling of despair. It is a morbid spirit of darkness. You give up and let the currents of despair wash away your personality. Your mind gets tired from constant pulling and tugging of your thoughts. You wake up tired having slept but not rested.

If we fail to tell the difference between common sadness and depression we may neglect a serious condition that requires treatment (depression) or, on the other end of the spectrum, overreact to a normal emotional state (sadness).

We know that depression is a very complex condition that can be rooted in spiritual, emotional, mental, biological, or physiological causes, or a combination thereof. If you struggle with depression, we hope you are seeking professional medical help. There is no shame in admitting that you need some assistance.

Pastor Rick Warren reminds people who suffer from mental illness that, "your illness is not your identity and your chemistry is not your character."[31]

Often, Christians add to their problems by feeling guilty because they are depressed. We must remove the stigma and shame of being mentally ill. Being sick isn't a sin and neither is living with mental illness.

In Psalm 77 we read of some possible causes for depression:-

- A morbid, pessimistic outlook on life can be a trigger for a depressive episode. *"In the day of my trouble I sought the Lord: my sore ran in the night, and ceased not: my soul refused to be comforted."* *(Psalm 77:2)* Some people are full of pessimism and are always thinking and speaking in the negative. As Christians we should cultivate a holy optimism and deliberately refuse to dwell upon the dark side of things.

- An offending conscience can lead to depression. *"I remembered God, and was troubled: ..." (Psalm 77:3a)*. In his depression he suddenly remembered God and was troubled. Evidently he did not have a conscience "void of offence". There was something between him and God.

---

31 http://www.azquotes.com/quote/868409

- A complaining spirit may produce thoughts leading to depression. *"... I complained, and my spirit was overwhelmed. Selah." (Psalm 77:3b).* The person who is always complaining is especially prone to depression.

- Dwelling on the past and living in regrets and unmet expectations can become depressive. *"I have considered the days of old, the years of ancient times." (Psalm 77:5)* To continually look back and focus on the 'should've, could've, would've, if only moments of life' can be a spring board into discouragement and ultimately depression.

- Too much unhealthy introspection can become a reason for depression. *"I call to remembrance my song in the night: I commune with mine own heart: and my spirit made diligent search." (Psalm 77:6)* We must make sure that our depression is not caused by sin. We do need to search and try our ways. However, we must at all cost avoid plunging into an unhealthy, unspiritual, morbid introspection that keeps looking inside and can see nothing but bad. Many of God's people are spiritually, mentally and physically ill because they keep looking at themselves.

- Leaving God out of our reckoning in our lives may be a reason why we are depressed. *"Will the Lord cast off for ever? and will he be favourable no more? Is his mercy clean gone for ever? doth his promise fail for evermore? Hath God forgotten to be gracious? hath he in anger shut up his tender mercies? Selah." (Psalm 77:7-9)* This is the all-inclusive reason we stay depressed. We fail to reckon on the presence, power and provision of our Lord and Saviour, Jesus Christ.

As a couple, we have personally classified depression into four categories:

Circumstantial depression – This is a response to the pain and trauma of living in a fallen world. It is a general depression caused by a loss, such as the death of a loved one or a tragic circumstance that has clearly become the source of the feeling of sadness and loss of interest. Exhaustion, broken relationships, family problems, divorce, pressure to excel in sports and school, work related factors, job loss, sickness, hormonal changes, postnatal fatigue, alcohol and drug abuse, even certain times of the year – winter, Christmas, anniversaries - can all bring on depression in a person. Men are seven times more likely to suffer from circumstantial depression than women. Most women have someone to talk things out with and their depression usually stems from the loss of a loved one, hormonal changes or physical sickness. Men, however, usually suffer from depression due to some social humiliation. They feel like a failure, they view themselves as a loser. They no longer feel like a man in a world of men. Instead of taking care of others, they need to be taken care of. Instead of providing, they feel like they are being provided for. It attacks their pride, it attacks their manhood and they respond in depression. This form of depression may require some counselling, psychotherapy, rest and refocus. Since our emotions respond to what we are thinking, circumstantial depression is most often the consequence of negative thinking about ourselves, our circumstances, others and even God. By honestly relating to God, He can correct our misbeliefs and renew our minds with His truth. Generally, this type of depression clears with counselling and/or time, as the circumstances are resolved or accepted. At times, some anti-depressant medication may be prescribed for the short-term depending on the individual situation to relax the body and relieve the mind to deal with the circumstances calmly and clearly.

Carnal depression – While this type of depression is not officially classified by mental health professionals, we have simply added it here to extend the classification of circumstantial depression, because we believe this type of depression definitely requires spiritual treatment not just counselling and/or medication. Some circumstantial depression is simply due to non-sinful events and circumstances of life. However, there is a depression that has been directly caused by sin, guilt, resentment, bitterness, grudges and wrong thinking in our fleshly (carnal) minds. The apostle Paul wrote, *"For to be carnally minded is death; but to be spiritually minded is life and peace. Because the carnal mind is enmity against God: for it is not subject to the law of God, neither indeed can be." (Romans 8:6-7)* This type of depression should be dealt with by confession, repentance and renewal of the mind. If a person has been living carnally and indulging in anger, self-centeredness and other sinful behaviours, this can be the reason they have sunk into depression. Circumstantial, yes, but nonetheless rooted in carnality. Sin always has negative consequences and part of any therapy for depression should include an analysis of what sins could be exacerbating the situation. In doing so this will help define whether the depression is merely circumstantial or whether it is carnally based. Being depressed is not a sin; it is more accurate to say that sometimes sin leads to and feeds depression. However, one is still accountable for the response to the affliction, including getting the spiritual and professional help that is needed.

Clinical depression – This depression is often said to be caused by a chemical imbalance in the brain and is what most drug treatments are based on. Certainly in many cases, there is a reduction in the amount of certain neurotransmitters (serotonin) found in depressed people. Any disruption to the physical processes of the brain can lead to chemical imbalances within the nervous system thereby leading to depression. Thyroid disorder, hypoglycaemia (low blood sugar), hormone imbalances in blood levels of estrogen and adrenaline, viral infections (flu, mononucleosis), vitamin shortages and premenstrual syndrome (PMS) can be contributing factors. Major depressive episodes are characteristic of both major depressive disorder (unipolar) and bipolar disorder. Most people suffering with bipolar will be diagnosed with a chemical imbalance. This type of depression is going to need some medical treatment and counselling tailored to the individuals health needs. If your body doesn't produce insulin naturally to break down sugars you think nothing of it. You are now chemically supplying what the body is not supplying. If your hypertension is not regulated properly and your blood pressure is high and you are endangering your heart – you control it with medicine. But when something is not secreting in your head, are you supposed to just pray about it? When your brain has a chemical imbalance you may need some help to balance it not just pray about it. Have you ever seen a dirty algae-infested swimming pool? When algae, dirt and fungus start to build up inside a swimming pool that means there is a chemical imbalance in the pool. The only way that you can treat an imbalance is to shock it with a dose of chlorine. Just like a pool has its chemicals way out of balance sometimes, so too can people. It's called serotonin levels. In the brain of a bipolar sufferer, the neurotransmitter (serotonin) gets muddy. What some people need to do is take medication to clear up their brain and they can see things a lot clearer. There is a depression that is chemical-treated.[32] Mental health researchers know something is awry in someone's brain when he/she shows symptoms of bipolar disorder and persistent depression and they know chemicals often can help alleviate these symptoms.[33]

32 http://www.medicaldaily.com/scientists-prove-chemical-imbalance-theory-schizophrenia-using-brain-model-made-stem-cells-302596
33 http://www.peteeearley.com/2015/01/30/mental-illnesses-caused-chemical-imbalances/

Chronic depression – This depression is less intense than clinical depression but can last much longer. A chronic form of depression, dysthymia is characterised by depressed mood on most days for at least two years. It's characterised by fatigue and sadness and it can be punctuated by bouts of clinical depression. While chronic depression doesn't feel good, it doesn't typically affect lifestyle or the ability to work. On some days individuals may feel relatively fine or even have moments of joy. But the good mood usually lasts no longer than a few weeks to a few months.

One thing is certain: as Christians, we have divine resources available that the world cannot use or even understand. When non-Christian people are depressed, they often resort to various means of escape - drugs, alcohol, sex, entertainment - but then discover that they have not really escaped themselves. When the show is over, or the 'high' is ended, they are worse off than before.

An encouraging and helpful psalm in the Bible that gives great advice for beating the blues and coming out of a depressive mood is Psalm 42. The psalmist's own experience of depression describes how he felt and also what he did about it. This song talks about those days when we feel like curling up in the foetal position and quitting! It talks about how we can conquer feelings of quitting rather than succumbing to them.

We really do not know who wrote this very personal psalm, but, whoever he was, he certainly was displaying signs of depression. We do not know if his depression would be classified as circumstantial, carnal or even clinical. What is important is that the psalm helps point the way to victory over the negative and damaging emotions flowing from depressive episodes.

Psalms are songs of hope written to awaken, express and shape the emotional life of God's people. Poetry and singing exist because God made us with emotions, not just thoughts. Our emotions are massively important. I (Jenny) have found immense comfort from reading through the psalms.

If you're looking for a way to beat the blues, Psalm 42 gives us three stops and three starts. If you want to overcome depression, then you must make some radical changes in your outlook on life. What do you need to stop and start?

STOP LOOKING AT YOURSELF AND START LOOKING AT GOD

"As the hart panteth after the water brooks, so panteth my soul after thee, O God. My soul thirsteth for God, for the living God: when shall I come and appear before God? My tears have been my meat day and night, while they continually say unto me, Where is thy God? When I remember these things, I pour out my soul in me: for I had gone with the multitude, I went with them to the house of God, with the voice of joy and praise, with a multitude that kept holyday." (Psalm 42:1-4)

The psalmist describes the inner thirst, the emptiness he feels. Just like a deer pants, longing for water – so too do we. Have you ever been that thirsty spiritually? Does your soul pant for God? David once spoke of this longing, *"O, God, thou art my God; early will I seek thee: my soul thirsteth for thee, my flesh longeth for thee in a dry and thirsty land, where no water is;" (Psalm 63:1)* Our longing for God cannot be satisfied by anything else.

The pop-star Madonna, when asked the question, "Are you a happy person?" replied, "I'm a tormented person. I have a lot of demons I'm wrestling with. But I want to be happy. I have moments of happiness. I'm working toward knowing myself... assuming that will bring me happiness."

Comedian Eddie Murphy told People magazine, "I feel something's missing...I don't think there's anyone who feels like there isn't something missing in their life. No matter how much money you make, or how many cars or houses you have, or how many people you make happy, life isn't perfect for anybody."

Jesus encountered a woman at the well of Samaria who tried to fill the longing in her heart with relationships with men. In fact she had a steady stream of broken relationships (she went through 5 husbands). She was living an empty life of shame. One day she went to a well to draw water at a time when no one else would be around. She met Jesus – The Well sitting on a well! Jesus said to her, "...*Whosoever drinketh of this water shall thirst again: But whosoever drinketh of the water that I shall give him shall never thirst; but the water that I shall give him shall be in him a well of water springing up into everlasting life.*" *(John 4:13-14)* In effect Jesus was saying, "Your thirst has been misplaced; the answer to your soul's thirst is me." When you're in a 'low' and depressed, it is not uncommon to cry a lot.

In the psalm the writer's appetite has vanished because of all his afflictions. His only source of nutrition is the salt from his own tears. He was 'feeding on tears' instead of eating his meals. He had fallen into the state of being so sorry for himself that he was feeding on his unfortunate situation. This led him deeper into depression. There was no relief. Day and night he cried. Hour after hour he succumbed to his feelings. There appeared to be no way out of his predicament. People hadn't helped much either. Some of them had taken the opportunity to kick him while he was down. It is bad enough being out of touch with the Lord, but it is ten times worse when people notice it and start to mock you.

His mind was fixed on his sorrows. Over and over he dwelt on the dismal disappointments of his life until he could think of nothing else. In the dark low times I (Jenny) have been the victim of negative thought patterns and saw myself spiralling further down into a dark abyss of depression. Often in times of depression I recall the 'good old days' as if they were fading memories and wonder if I will ever have another opportunity to enjoy them. I feel like the psalmist brooding alone in my misery.

These are the classic symptoms of depression: Self-pity, brooding, withdrawal, morbid reminiscing and introspection. When I am in the blues and despair of depression, I have sought to follow the lessons from this psalm and stop looking at myself and start looking to God.

In the first four verses of Psalm 42 there are twelve personal pronouns – 'me, my, I' and there are six references to 'God.' We get the impression that the writer was looking primarily at himself. It is a dangerous thing to look at yourself too much. I (Robert) have noticed over the years that when Jenny would swing to a low mood her introspection became very negative. Even as she would look at the Bible, her focus would always be drawn to the sad and morbid aspects of the scriptures and overlook the antidote verses of joy, peace, hope and love.

In depression we end up seeing ourselves no matter where we look. This explains why a change in circumstances cannot of itself cure depression: we take our hearts with us. It is natural for us to think mainly of ourselves when we are going through difficult times. We must constantly remind ourselves to walk by faith and to see God in the picture. After all, God is in control of this universe!

If we are truly thirsting after God and not just His help and deliverance, then the experience that could tear us down will actually build us up. Instead of complaining, we will be praying and praising God. Life will not be a mirror in which we see only ourselves; it will be a window through which we see God.

At the end of this section of Psalm 42, David recalls the power of *"the voice of joy and praise."* He already knows that depression and heaviness of soul will deplete a person of emotional and physical strength. *"My soul melteth for heaviness: strengthen thou me according unto thy word." (Psalm 119:28)* However, praise will empower and replenish a worshipper. When we begin to praise the Lord for Who He is and What He has done and can do, whether it be through song or prayer, then it's amazing what praising can do. Isaiah, the Old Testament prophet, reminds the person who feels weighed down in spirit to lighten their load through praise. *"To appoint unto them that mourn in Zion, to give unto them beauty for ashes, the oil of joy for mourning, **the garment of praise for the spirit of heaviness**; that they might be called trees of righteousness, the planting of the LORD, that he might be glorified." (Isaiah 61:3)* Nothing jump starts the spirit like praise. The single most powerful, medicinal tool to help the spirit of heaviness is praise.

STOP LOOKING BACK AND START LOOKING FORWARD

*"**Why** art thou cast down, O my soul? and **why** art thou disquieted in me? hope thou in God: for I shall yet praise him for the help of his*

countenance. O my God, my soul is cast down within me: therefore will I remember thee from the land of Jordan, and of the Hermonites, from the hill Mizar. Deep calleth unto deep at the noise of thy waterspouts: all thy waves and thy billows are gone over me. Yet the LORD will command his lovingkindness in the daytime, and in the night his song shall be with me, and my prayer unto the God of my life. I will say unto God my rock, **Why** *hast thou forgotten me?* **why** *go I mourning because of the oppression of the enemy? As with a sword in my bones, mine enemies reproach me; while they say daily unto me, Where is thy God? (Psalm 42:5-10)*

I (Jenny) have found it a common occurrence to question why I was the way I was. I think it is a normal human tendency to want an answer or explanation for the illness or malady we may suffer.

In fact there may well be reasons why we have fallen into a state of depression. The psalmist asks *"why"* four times in these verses. He started to look back and wonder what happened. We have found it helpful to do a little detective work to try to discover if there had been any triggers that may have given rise to the onset of a bipolar episode.

By delving into our own situation and asking some pertinent questions, we can start to determine if this depression is circumstantial, carnal or clinical. The psalmist asks his soul, *"Why art thou cast down, O my soul? and why art thou disquieted in me?"* His question is factual and pertinent. "Why are you depressed, soul?"

This question, if handled honestly, may lead the depressed person into some deep and convicting personal discoveries. You might find yourself filled with resentment, anger towards God, bitterness and/or fear. These emotions and attitudes may very well be what has brought about the circumstantial or carnal depression.

To move forward you have to admit – "I'm cast down, I am actually disquieted within me." The psalmist was realistic enough to admit that he was depressed. Sometimes it is easier to dwell on your unfortunate circumstances in which you find yourself. But it's your condition, not your circumstances, that is really important.

If a man gets shot in the leg, there are two courses he could follow. He could sit down and ponder the fact that he got shot, take photographs of his wound, study books on ballistics and take a course in the psychological abnormalities of potential assassins. Or he could say, "I'm shot. Get me to the doctor!" For some people who are suffering with depression, they simply need to admit it and get some help.

We need to bring the Lord into the depression in our life. Give your soul a good talking to. "Listen to me, Soul. - You have been *disquieted within me*' far too long. It's time for something different. 'Hope thou in God'. Now that's an order!"

We have a choice to make – Go toward God or not? When you're in the pits and you feel like there's no way out, then resolve to remember what is true. I (Jenny) know that when I'm down, it's easy for me to lose sight of what is really true. Doubts can creep in and despair can skewer my soul. Even though I know what is true, I need to force myself to remember it or I will have a difficult time overcoming the blues.

Notice the shift in thinking, *"Why art thou cast down, O my soul? and why art thou disquieted in me?* **hope thou in God**: *for **I shall yet praise him** for the help of his countenance."* (Psalm 42:5) Remind yourself to hope in God and tell yourself you will praise God again. Tell yourself God is smiling on you – He is your helper. The thought is that God's face is never marked by disappointment. When He looks upon us, it is with love and mercy. The best solution to depression and disappointment is to see the face of God as He smiles upon us.

People who are depressed are often living in the past. But people who conquer depression are those who live in the future. If memories of pain and hurt dominate your thought life it is because those memories have your attention. How can a memory hurt you? The event has already happened and it can only hurt you if it has your attention. If you turn your attention from the memory of the past you will take away the power from the pain or hurt. You may need counselling to help with processing hurts, bitterness and other issues from the past but you can trust the same God who has never failed or forsaken you. God does care for you – that is without question. *"Yet the LORD will command his lovingkindness in the daytime, and in the night his song shall be with me, and my prayer unto the God of my life."* (Psalm 42:8)

How do we pray to *"the God of my life"* whilst we are in depression? We can follow the pattern of the psalmist.

- Pray **heartily** (from your heart) – *"my prayer"*. Don't be afraid to sing, cry, or laugh.

- Pray **humbly** to *"the God of my life."* He is God. Come before Him with a sense of awe in His presence.

- Pray **honestly** – He knows what you're going through (just be honest about how you feel). It is normal for us to ask questions when we are hurting or going through perplexing experiences. It is not wrong to ask questions of God, but it is wrong to question God. Our attitude should be one of submissive concern and not rebellious complaint.

David talked about *"God my rock"*. Now that's the sort of thing a depressed person should meditate on. When all seems lost and you have an awful sinking feeling, what could be better than to know that there is a rock beneath you upon which you can stand when you're sinking?

STOP LOOKING FOR WHY AND START LOOKING TO WHOM

"Why art thou cast down, O my soul? and why art thou disquieted within me? hope thou in God: for I shall yet praise him, who is the health of my countenance, and my God." (Psalm 42:11)

There are nine questions asked in Psalm 42. Six times the psalmist asked *"why?"* and we have no record that God ever gave him an answer. God never told him WHY he had depression. Suppose God had answered all his questions; would that have solved any problems and made him feel any better? No! It is a basic fact of life that we do not live on explanations; we live on promises. We must stop searching for reasons and start resting on promises.

If you were to break a leg and then go to a hospital for help, medical professionals would x-ray the leg and study the break in the bone. On the basis of that study, the doctor would set the broken bone and put your leg in a cast. If the doctor came into your room with the x-rays and carefully explained how the bone was broken and what he did to repair it, would that make you feel any better? Maybe. But if the doctor said, "You will be out of the cast and walking again in eight weeks", that would encourage you. We live on promises, not explanations. An explanation may satisfy the curiosity of the mind, but only a promise can heal the hurt in the heart and give strength to the will.

Even if God did give reasons for all His acts, we would not be satisfied. In fact, it would be impossible for us to fully understand all that God is doing. We walk by faith, not by sight or by explanations.

The answer for WHY questions is WHOM. That answer to life's problems is not a program or a prescription or possessions, but a Person – God Himself.

I (Robert) preached a sermon once on how to become depressed in five easy steps. The message focused on the life of Elijah the prophet and his depression and suicidal disposition in 1 Kings 19. The fives steps identified in this chapter were:

- Fatigue - Wear yourself out.
- Fear - Let your worries consume your thinking.
- Flee - Shut friends and people out.
- Focus – Think on the negative.
- Forget – Don't remember the faithfulness of God.

It's this last step that can be addressed in every depressed Christian's life. We must focus back on the WHOM and stop looking for the WHY.

Sadly, many try to self medicate in an attempt to rid themselves of the gnawing pain of depression. Some self medicate with sleeping pills so that they don't have to deal with it. Others throw themselves into their career and work harder and harder. We have known of people who self medicate with sarcasm, so they can kind of laugh their way through life. Solomon, the writer of proverbs, had identified people like this and said, *"Even in laughter the heart is sorrowful; and the end of that mirth is heaviness."* *(Proverbs 14:13)* The internet, social media, drugs, alcohol, sex and entertainment are often relied upon in an attempt to numb the ache in the soul. I am so glad that the real healing for the noisy soul is God. He is the healer of the hearts. *"He healeth the broken in heart, and bindeth up their wounds."* *(Psalm 147:3)*

When something is broken it doesn't work properly, but God is the One who can heal the broken things of life. He's the healer. If it's anxiety, if it's worry, if it's fear, if you have thought about suicide, if you are lonely…the list goes on. We want you to know that Jesus Christ is the surgeon of your soul. He wants to so delicately heal your wounds. He will give you a peace that passes all understanding.

There is no doubt that a depressed person often shows on his face what is going on inside his head. But the Lord can make all the difference. He can put a smile on your face and help you beat the blues.

CHAPTER 16

FEAR NOT

DREAD

Shohoiya Yokowai spent 28 years of his life in prison. It was not a prison of iron bars, locks and jail wardens, but a self-imposed prison of fear. He was a Japanese soldier on the island of Guam during World War II and when the American forces landed, he fled into the jungle and found a cave. He hid in the cave for 28 years because he was afraid of being captured by the Americans. He learned that the war was over by reading one of the thousands of pamphlets dropped into the jungle from American airplanes, but he was still afraid. So for 28 years he lived in the cave coming out only at night to look for cockroaches, rats, frogs and mangoes on which he survived. Finally some natives found him and convinced him that it would be all right for him to come out of his jungle prison.

When we hear of stories like this we think, "What a waste! Imagine spending 28 years living as a prisoner of fear." Yet, there are a lot of people who are prisoners of fear every day of their life. This is a common feature of bipolar sufferers.

When I (Jenny) first began to experience the symptoms of bipolar disorder, though at that stage did not know what was wrong with me, fear of the unknown consumed me. A former pastor counselled with me about the issue of fear and suggested that the reason I was feeling so low had everything to do with my fears.

I began to memorise and meditate on verses of scripture concerning fear, like *"What time I am afraid, I will trust in thee. In God I will praise his word, in God I have put my trust; I will not fear what flesh can do unto me." (Psalm 56:3-4)*. Another verse I would cling to reminded me of the power of God and His protection, *"Fear ye not, neither be afraid: have not I told thee from that time, and have declared it? ye are even my witnesses. Is there a God beside me? yea, there is no God; I know not any." (Isaiah 44:8)*

Many are held as prisoners because of fear. Fear is very much a part of our lives and there is nobody who is exempt from having this emotion.

Some may be afraid of losing a job, or their health, or losing finances. Others may be fearful of not being accepted by others, or be just afraid of growing old. The list could go on and on.

As a result, we try to take precautions to protect ourselves. We buy insurance policies to cover those things we consider valuable. We put bars on our windows and locks on our doors and install alarm systems to protect our homes, businesses and automobiles. Whilst some of these measures are prudent common sense, they are nonetheless driven by fear of loss.

There are several types of fear:

- *Healthy Fear* keeps us from avoiding dangerous situations, such as respecting electricity, fire or turning the gas off when we smell a leak. Fear is a God-given emotion that prepares our body and mind to deal with challenges in life. There is nothing wrong with having fear in such instances. In fact, it can be a very healthy emotion to have. It can help save your life.

- *Harmful Fear* paralyses us. It keeps us from doing things we could or should do. Satan is a master at using our fears. Fear is one of his primary weapons to cause panic, confusion and chaos. Satan uses common fears of failure and rejection to cause many people to never start or try anything and to make Christians ineffective in their witness.

Our fear of failure can cause us to put things off. We do everything we can to avoid facing the possibility of messing up, as in the parable of the talents that Jesus gave. *"Then he which had received the one talent came and said, Lord, I knew thee that thou art an hard man, reaping where thou hast not sown, and gathering where thou hast not strawed: And **I was afraid**, and went **and hid** thy talent in the earth: lo, there thou hast that is thine."* (Matthew 25:24-25) In the parable this man buried his talent and exposed his fear, when he should have buried his fear and exposed his talent. Fear paralysed him from using his initiative and taking action.

Fear of rejection makes us afraid to do anything that could draw criticism or shame, or give someone a chance to laugh at us. This is the fear the first man Adam had after he had sinned. *"And he said, I heard thy voice in the garden, and I was afraid, because I was naked; and **I hid myself."** (Genesis 3:10)* Fear causes people to cover up and hide behind excuses, lies, false imaginations, escape plans and many other forms of self-protection.

- *Hurtful Fear* is uncontrolled fear and is destructive. This is when the fear becomes a torture to the mind and destroys and debilitates the person. This is where people can have panic attacks and suffer terrible anxiety disorders. For sufferers of bipolar and other mental illnesses, this type of fear is very prevalent. In the 'low' episodes I (Jenny) have found I can become more vulnerable to hurtful fears through intrusive and unwanted thoughts that can easily trigger anxiety. It is not that the fears have been the triggers to push me into depression; rather it is when the low hits me and depression overwhelms my mind, it is then that fears start to dominate my thinking. Panic plagues my mind if I allow myself to dwell on my fearful thoughts of losing control. I have had panic attacks in the past. I would get sudden feelings of terror, heart palpitations, breathing difficulties, nausea and dizziness whilst being swamped with feelings of doom. Early on in my illness it was not uncommon for me to hyper-ventilate during one of these episodes. I learned to carry a brown paper bag with me to help with my breathing and avoid hyper-ventilating.

Dr Walter Cannon, a pioneer researcher in psychosomatic medicine at Harvard University, describes what happens to the human body when it becomes angry or fearful: *"Respiration deepens; the heart beats more rapidly; the arterial pressure rises; the blood is shifted from the stomach and intestines to the heart, central nervous system, and the muscles; the processes of the alimentary canal cease; sugar is freed from the reserves in the liver; the spleen contracts and discharges its contents of concentrated corpuscles, and adrenalin is secreted."* It is little wonder a person feels nauseated with all this happening inside them.

When anxiety controlled by fear strikes your life it affects the mind. The apostle Paul recognised this and reminds us in the scriptures that this is not God's desire. *"For God hath not given us the spirit of fear; but of power, and of love, and of a sound mind." (2 Timothy 1:7)*

When fear is dominating my thinking, the thought patterns generally go like this:

- I experience lack of enthusiasm and just know I am going to fail. Life is no longer exciting and purposeful.

- My thoughts become unfocused and all I can think about is what I fear – being out of control.

- My fear and anxiety keep me from interacting with others and all I want to do is to be alone.

- Being consumed by fear keeps me from getting anything done. I tend to procrastinate because I can't think straight.

- At times I feel I'm a terrible Christian and have even blamed God for causing my problems.

- I generally overstate and magnify problems and minimise what God and His Word state is possible. Fear brings God's promises to naught.

- In an anxious state I have an inability to cope with even small problems.

- Decision-making becomes difficult (both major and minor kinds).

- I can have sudden outbursts of temper and hostility and verbally attack Robert.

- Forgetfulness occurs for appointments, deadlines and important dates.

Probably the worst thing about fear is the worry it produces and worry does nothing but make matters worse in our minds. An average person's anxiety is focused on:

- 40% on things that will probably never happen.

- 30% on things about the past that can't be changed.

- 12% on things about criticism by others, mostly untrue.

- 10% about health, which gets worse with stress.

- 8% about real problems that will be faced.

Anxiety adds distress to our difficulties and only creates more problems. Our anxiety adds additional stress to our lives. Pastor Adrian Rogers once said, *"Worry pulls tomorrow's cloud over today's sunshine."*[34]

Worry is relative to each of our situations and it's not an easy thing to just stop worrying. Worry is based in fear and we all have many fears. There are almost 200 categories of phobias that can crawl over us like ants on a picnic lunch.

I (Robert) read a book written by comedian Jerry Seinfeld called "SeinLanguage", where he spoke about fear. He said, *"According to most studies, people's number one fear is public speaking. Number two is death. Death is number two. Does that seem right? That means to the average person, if you have to go to a funeral, you're better off in the coffin than doing the eulogy."*[35]

In 1988 Bobby McFerrin wrote a song called *"Don't Worry, Be happy."* The lyrics hone in on the futility of worry.

---

34 http://www.oneplace.com/ministries/love-worth-finding/read/articles/a-word-for-worriers-9900.html
35 http://www.goodreads.com/quotes/162599

Here is a little song I wrote
You might want to sing it note for note
Don't worry be happy
In every life we have some trouble
When you worry you make it double
Don't worry, be happy...

Have you ever had those words said to you? Did it work? They are easy words to say, but hard to put into practice.

You can worry yourself to death, but not to life. Dr Charles Mayo, of the famous Mayo Clinic, wrote, *"Worry affects the circulation, the heart, the glands and the whole nervous system. I have never met a man or known a man to die of overwork, but I have known a lot who died of worry."*[36]

The English word 'worry' comes from an old German word meaning "to strangle, or choke". Worry is mental and emotional strangulation.

The more you worry, the more it slows you down. Worry produces heaviness in the heart of man. *"Heaviness in the heart of man maketh it stoop: but a good word maketh it glad."* (Proverbs 12:25) You don't feel light when you worry. You feel heavy. You feel pressed down. You feel depressed. Worry weighs a person down.

Worry exhausts your energy and you get worn out. *"I am weary with my groaning; all the night make I my bed to swim; I water my couch with my tears."* (Psalm 6:6). Worry actually drains energy out of you and saps your strength. It exhausts you.

Worry exaggerates a problem. You start worrying about something and it gets bigger and bigger in your mind. *"The troubles of my heart* are enlarged: O bring thou me out of my distresses." (Psalm 25:17) Worry is an irrational, illogical form of thought. It makes your problems bigger, not smaller. Little fears turn into big fears.

Holocaust survivor Corrie Ten Boom said, "*Worrying is carrying tomorrow's load with today's strength - carrying two days at once. It is moving into tomorrow ahead of time. Worrying doesn't empty tomorrow of its sorrow, it empties today of its strength.*"[37]

Jesus spoke about the futility of worry and fear. He dealt with three common worries amongst people - what shall we eat? what shall we drink? and what shall we wear? Jesus' response is, "Don't give it a second thought." People in Jesus' day worried about the necessities of life: food, drink and clothing. Today in the Western world we worry about other things, such as cancer, terrorism, losing our jobs, our children's safety and, we worry about our illnesses. Jesus' words apply to our worries as well.

Jesus said worry is **unreasonable** – "*Therefore I say unto you, Take no thought for your life, what ye shall eat, or what ye shall drink; nor yet for your body, what ye shall put on. Is not the life more than meat, and the body than raiment?*" (Matthew 6:25)

Jesus said worry is **unnatural** – "*Behold the fowls of the air: for they sow not, neither do they reap, nor gather into barns; yet your heavenly Father feedeth them. Are ye not much better than they?*" (Matthew 6:26) Don't ever assume that God doesn't care about you. He says you are "*much better*" than His creation. It's as if Jesus says in this verse, "Have you forgotten who your Father is?" If God feeds the birds of the air will He not provide for you? He cares about you much more than He cares about birds. At times we can accuse God

---

37 http://www.goodreads.com/quotes/110765-worrying-is-carrying-tomorrow-s-load-with-today-s-strength--carrying-two

of not caring for us because we have already decided what His care for us should be. We have already mapped out in our minds how we think God should work. We think things like, "Where are you God?" or "God, I don't understand how you would let this happen to me." I (Jenny) have said, "God, you're good and all, but I'm struggling here. What if I don't make it?"

Jesus said worry is **unhelpful** – *"Which of you by taking thought can add one cubit unto his stature?" (Matthew 6:27)* Worry does not change anything. Worry has never solved any problem in the history of the human race. So it's just a worthless waste of energy and thought and emotion.

Jesus said worry is **unnecessary** – *"And why take ye thought for raiment? Consider the lilies of the field, how they grow; they toil not, neither do they spin: And yet I say unto you, That even Solomon in all his glory was not arrayed like one of these. Wherefore, if God so clothe the grass of the field, which to day is, and to morrow is cast into the oven, shall he not much more clothe you, O ye of **little faith**?"* (Matthew 6:28-30) Jesus concluded by challenging us all on the issue of faith in God. Fear and faith cannot exist in the same heart at the same time. Faith is what will conquer our fears.

> *Fear imprisons but faith liberates.*
> *Fear paralyses but faith empowers.*
> *Fear disheartens but faith encourages.*
> *Fear sickens but faith heals.*
> *Fear makes useless but faith makes useful.*
> *Fear puts hopelessness at the heart of life, while faith rejoices in its God.*[38]

---

38 "Another One Bites the Dust" By Malcolm White, Gospel Folio Press, 2010, page 78

The answer to our worrying and fearfulness is to guard our thought life and place our faith and trust in our Heavenly Father to care for us and love us. *"Therefore take no thought, saying, What shall we eat? or, What shall we drink? or, Wherewithal shall we be clothed? (For after all these things do the Gentiles seek:) for your heavenly Father knoweth that ye have need of all these things. But seek ye first the kingdom of God, and his righteousness; and all these things shall be added unto you. Take therefore no thought for the morrow: for the morrow shall take thought for the things of itself. Sufficient unto the day is the evil thereof."* (Matthew 6:31-34)

Have you ever lain in bed tossing and turning, with all kinds of thoughts running through your mind? An unchecked thought life is lethal to the Christian life. We need to guard what enters our minds. Stop magnifying problems and minimizing God. Start magnifying God and minimizing the problems. As Christians we have a Heavenly Father who loves us and values us more than anything else in the world. He cares for us.

When we worry, we stop trusting God and start trying to take control of our own life. Sometimes we forget that God is not only in control of our lives, but He's also in control of this entire universe. If God can handle every single thing in this world, He can handle everything in our life.

The apostle Peter encourages us to take our worries and cares to the Lord. *"Casting all your care upon him; for he careth for you."* (1 Peter 5:7) Remember that God cares for us. Why is this important to remember? Because there are times when we will wonder if anybody cares about what we are going through.

The psalmist David draws our attention back to the Lord and confidently reminds us all, *"The LORD is my light and my salvation;*

whom shall I fear? *the LORD is the strength of my life; of* **whom shall I be afraid?**" *(Psalm 27:1)*

The song writer, Chris Tomlin, wrote a song entitled *"Whom shall I fear?"*[39] that captures the essence of this verse of Scripture and encourages us to live by faith and put our fear to flight.

> *You hear me when I call*
> *You are my morning song*
> *Though darkness fills the night*
> *It cannot hide the light*
> *Whom shall I fear*
> *You crush the enemy*
> *Underneath my feet*
> *You are my sword and shield*
> *Though troubles linger still*
> *Whom shall I fear*
> *I know who goes before me*
> *I know who stands behind*
> *The God of angel armies*
> *Is always by my side*
> *The one who reigns forever*
> *He is a friend of mine*
> *The God of angel armies*
> *Is always by my side*

The Bible gives us the prescription to overcome worry and care: it is through the avenue of prayer. When you pray and talk to the Lord it is like a pressure relief valve and allows you to cast your burden and cares upon Him. *"Be careful for nothing; but in every thing by prayer*

---

39 http://www.metrolyrics.com/whom-shall-i-fear-god-of-angel-armies-lyrics-chris-tomlin.html

and supplication with thanksgiving let your requests be made known unto God. And the peace of God, which passeth all understanding, shall keep your hearts and minds through Christ Jesus." (Philippians 4:6-7)

Tell the Lord the emotions you feel and have bottled up; pour out your soul to Him. Learn to thank God for the small mercies every day and confess to Him your lack of trust and faith. Ask the Lord to increase your faith and remove your fears. Cast your cares upon the Lord one by one. *"Cast thy burden upon the LORD, and he shall sustain thee: he shall never suffer the righteous to be moved." (Psalm 55:22)*

God is concerned about everything, so turn everything over to Him. He watches over us, just as he sees the sparrow fall and knows the number of hairs upon our head. *"Are not two sparrows sold for a farthing? and one of them shall not fall on the ground without your Father. But the very hairs of your head are all numbered. Fear ye not therefore, ye are of more value than many sparrows." (Matthew 10:29-31)*

There is a difference between being concerned about the future and worry. You can make the situation better by planning and evaluating, but not by worrying. There is nothing wrong with making preparations and taking precautions, but there is everything wrong with being worried. I (Jenny) had to come to the point in life when I realised my life is never out of control – it is always under His control.

Conquering worry and fear is not a matter of self-determination. It is a matter of dependence on God whom we can trust and LOVE. It is a matter of belief in His words, His promises and His gifts to you. It is a matter of recognizing the devils pitiful attempts at crippling you with fear and God's majestic grace in giving you power, LOVE and a sound mind.

Any person who has allowed fear to rule their heart and mind will know that fear has torment. That is, fear causes agony, pain, anguish, and misery. Fear and anxiety torture the soul, poison the mind, cripple the will, and harden the heart. Thankfully, the Bible teaches that perfect LOVE casts out fear. *"There is **no fear in love**; but **perfect love casteth out fear**: because **fear hath torment**. He that feareth is not made perfect in **love**."* *(1 John 4:18)* Just as fear and faith cannot co-exist, neither can fear and love. The closer you get to love the farther you get from fear, but the other side is true also. The closer you get to fear the farther you get from love. They are like the north pole and the south pole. The closer you get to one the farther you get from the other. The more you learn about the love of God and the more perfectly you love, the farther you drift from fear. Pastor Rick Warren said, "Fear is a self-imposed prison that will keep you from becoming what God intends for you to be. You must move against it with the weapons of faith and love."[40]

When Jesus was asked, "What is the greatest commandment?" He answered without hesitation. He said, *"And thou shalt **love** the Lord thy God with all thy heart, and with all thy soul, and with all thy mind, and with all thy strength: this is the first commandment."* *(Mark 12:30)*

What happens if I love God with my body, heart devotion, emotions and mind? That means I no longer need to be afraid of what can afflict me physically. I no longer need to be afraid of mental anxieties. I no longer need to be afraid of emotional insecurities - because *"perfect love casteth out fear."*

There is a story about a widow who had successfully raised a very large family and was being interviewed by a reporter. She had raised six of her own children and adopted twelve others. She always maintained stability and confidence. The reporter asked what her secret was, to

40 This quote is taken from the book "The Purpose Driven Life" by Rick Warren

which the woman said that she was in a partnership: "Many years ago I said, 'Lord, I'll do the works and you do the worrying.' And I haven't had an anxious care since."

CHAPTER 17

HOLD ON TO THE PROMISES

DESIRE

Florence Chadwick was the first woman to swim the English Channel both ways. On July 4, 1951, she was going to swim from Catalina to the California coastline. She didn't quite make it. It wasn't the cold waters. It wasn't the sharks. It wasn't the 15-16 hour swim. It was the fact that the fog rolled in and she couldn't see the coastline. She quit half a mile from the goal. When she got out of the water she said, "I'm not trying to make an excuse but I feel like if the fog hadn't been there and I could have seen the land, I would have made it." Later she tried again. The fog rolled in again but this time she knew that the coastline was there. And she completed the swim. In fact, she did it in two hours less time than anybody else had ever done it.

The fog of life has rolled in on most of our lives at some point in time. We either give up on our desires or we push ahead believing the coastline of our goal is still there. Just like the California coastline is immovable, so too the promises of God are immovable and you can rely on them during the fog of life. You may not be able to see them but it's hope that gives you the knowledge that they are there if you just go on. Sometimes when the fog rolls in, you feel behind and you feel like there's no hope, it's not true. Trust the fact that God is working in your life in the midst of your bipolar, or whatever your problem is, even though you can't see it.

Even though the diminishing of hope affects the emotions of the heart and mind, the key is to rekindle a desire within the bipolar victim. The wise words of King Solomon in the proverbs reminds us that, *"Hope deferred maketh the heart sick: but when the desire cometh, it is a tree of life." (Proverbs 13:12)* In other words even though it seemed your situation was hopeless, there is still a chance for change and that's why desire must not slip away.

In the New Testament, the word 'hope' occurs one time before the resurrection of Jesus, but it occurs sixty times after the resurrection. It doesn't take a genius to figure out where hope comes from. It comes from the resurrection. The resurrection started with a cross. Hope begins at the darkest places of our lives. If you want an illustration of how God sends problems into the world to bring good into the world, don't look any farther than the cross and the resurrection of Jesus Christ. The cross tells us that He not only understands our pain but He can transform our pain.

It is hope that enables someone who has been victimized in a terrible way to not only find healing in their life but have the ability to help someone else who's been victimized. It's hope that enables one who is just not sure about the future to put one foot in front of the other and keep going on, knowing that God has a future even though you don't know what it is. It is hope that enables someone to take a dream that has been shattered and watch God begin to put it together piece by piece one at a time. It's hope that enables you to look forward to the future even when you've sat down across the desk from that doctor and he has looked you in the eye and said, "It's not going to get any better." You know that there's a better day coming.

Hope in the Bible is not a wish. We go to the movies and say, "I hope this is going to be a good movie." We go through a drive-through thinking, "I hope I get what I ordered." I wish... I hope so... " When the Bible uses "hope", it doesn't mean "I wish"; it means it's a fact. It's a certainty.

It's not "I hope so…"

It's…

"I hope… so I have confidence."

"I hope … so I'm not afraid."

"I hope… so I can walk into the future."

Real hope to the soul is like oxygen to the body. You can't live without it. Hope is God's expected end. Hope is a confident expectation. *"For I know the thoughts that I think toward you, saith the LORD, thoughts of peace, and not of evil, to give you an expected end." (Jeremiah 29:11)*

There is a four-word definition of hope. Hope is when we realise that "God is in control." When we realise that God's plan will always prevail, we can have hope. He gives you an *"expected end"*.

The kind of hope that God gives changes everything. If we have the hope God wants us to have we can get started again. We can live with bipolar disorder. We can make it through. It is hope that enables us to handle tremendous pressure.

Hope is what gives us the strength to go on after a loss or a disappointment. In the previous chapter we spoke about discerning the voices. Do we listen to bipolar or do we listen to what hope says? In this chapter we want to look briefly at the last part of Romans 8. This is one of the greatest chapters in the Bible. It lists five promises that keep our hope up. It gives us the five benefits of being a believer.

If you've been feeling a little down or discouraged, these verses of scripture are bound to fill you with more hope.

Christians can always be hopeful because of these five simple truths.

GOD'S PURPOSE TRANSFORMS MY PROBLEMS

"And we know that all things work together for good to them that love God, to them who are the called according to his purpose. For whom he did foreknow, he also did predestinate to be conformed to the image of his Son, that he might be the firstborn among many brethren. Moreover whom he did predestinate, them he also called: and whom he called, them he also justified: and whom he justified, them he also glorified." (Romans 8:28-30)

I can always be hopeful because His purpose transforms my problems. God uses everything that happens in my life in a plan for my own good. Life is just a series of problems. For bipolar sufferers you may be in an episode right now as you read this book, or you are just coming out of an episode or you're headed into a new one. That's living with bipolar.

One of the most difficult kind of problems to hold on to or to understand are those that seem meaningless. You don't see a purpose in them. Why is this happening to me? It's not fair. When you don't understand a problem that's the most difficult kind to handle. But when you see a purpose behind the problem, when you see a meaning, when you see that there could be some kind of benefit from it that gives you a reason to hope. God has a purpose for every single problem you go through. No matter how big, no matter how little.

Many people misunderstand this verse. It does not say that all things are good. Cancer is not good. Rape is not good. Bankruptcy is not good. There are many bad things. In heaven everything is done perfectly. This is earth. We're fallen. It also does not say that all things work out the way we want them to. We'd like it to say that but it doesn't say that. It also does not say all things have a happy ending. On earth not all things have a happy ending. There are some very sad endings to things in life. But it does say, *"we know"*. That means we don't hope, we don't wish, we don't imagine, we don't desire, we don't guess. We have absolute confidence that what He's about to say is true. What do we know? – *"all things work together for good."* There is a grand design behind it all.

God causes all things to work together for good, including my bipolar. The *"things"* of my life God will *"work together"*. Not separately but together. We mentioned earlier that our life felt like a tapestry. The underside looks like a tangled mess. On the front side there's a beautiful picture. God is weaving a tapestry of your life into a beautiful picture. We look up and think, "God what are you doing with my life?" God replies, "Making all things work together for good." We just need to trust God in the process from start to finish. He's got the past, the present, the future all worked out. In the past He foreknew and predestined us. In the present He called and justified us. In the future we're going to be glorified.

GOD'S PROTECTION RELIEVES MY FEARS

"What shall we then say to these things? If God be for us, who can be against us?" (Romans 8:31)

Fear is another great cause of hopelessness. It is a very damaging, destructive emotion. Psychologists have identified 645 different fears. All people have fears in their life that plague them. When you are full of fear you cannot be full of hope. It pulls you down and it causes you to despair. Bipolar opens the door to fear and can have a crippling effect in your life if you let it. I'm thankful that God has placed the words, *"fear not"* 366 times in the Bible. One for every day of the year, even the leap year!

If you are a Christian, God is not only with you all the time but He is for you. If you read the last chapter of the Bible you will find out that you are on the winning side. We may lose a few battles here on earth while living with bipolar, but ultimately we win.

God is greater than anything life throws at you.

GOD'S PROVISION WILL SUPPLY MY NEEDS

"He that spared not his own Son, but delivered him up for us all, how shall he not with him also freely give us all things?" (Romans 8:32)

God has promised to meet every single need in your life if you'll trust Him. He'll meet your emotional, physical, spiritual, mental, relational and social needs. If God loves us enough to send Christ to die for us doesn't He care enough to take care of all our other needs? He has promised to take care of any other need if you put Him first in that area of your life. God wants to bless your life. *"For the LORD God is a sun and shield: the LORD will give grace and glory: no good thing will he withhold from them that walk uprightly." (Psalm 84:11)*

GOD'S PARDON SETS ME FREE

"Who shall lay any thing to the charge of God's elect? It is God that justifieth. Who is he that condemneth? It is Christ that died, yea rather, that is risen again, who is even at the right hand of God, who also maketh intercession for us." (Romans 8:33-34)

Sometimes, in a bipolar state I feel guilty and condemned. What do I do when I feel so guilty in my life? How could God love me, when I'm so unworthy of His love? He sees my life … knows how I live … knows me inside and out … knows when I fail Him and fail to live up to His love. Paul answers that question. When God accepts you for who and what you are and loves you anyhow … who else's opinion matters? People might criticise you, condemn you, gossip about you, cheat you, find fault and nit-pick about you, berate or belittle you or accuse you. Who dares accuse us now? The Judge Himself has declared us free from sin. Who is in a position to condemn? Only Christ and Christ died for us, Christ rose for us, Christ reigns in power for us and He prays for us.

God loves you so much that nobody else's opinion matters but His. I don't ever have to worry about any accusation from God. He's not accusing me. He's not against me, He's for me. Since He died and paid the price, no one else has the right, or the power to judge you and me.

GOD'S PROMISE SECURES MY FUTURE

"Who shall separate us from the love of Christ? shall tribulation, or distress, or persecution, or famine, or nakedness, or peril, or sword? As it is written, For thy sake we are killed all the day long; we are

accounted as sheep for the slaughter. Nay, in all these things we are more than conquerors through him that loved us. For I am persuaded, that neither death, nor life, nor angels, nor principalities, nor powers, nor things present, nor things to come, Nor height, nor depth, nor any other creature, shall be able to separate us from the love of God, which is in Christ Jesus our Lord." (Romans 8:35-39)

When Jesus took on our sin, died on the cross, was buried in a tomb and arose on the third day, He conquered sin, death and the grave. That's why Paul says that we are more than conquerors because the conquest has been completed. God will never ever stop loving me. Nothing can destroy my relationship with God. It doesn't matter how I feel, how many doubts, how many fears, or how many sins I commit, if I have put my trust in Christ, He says nothing will separate me from the love of God.

If you feel far from God, guess who moved?

God could never love you any more than He already does. With this I can find hope to cope.

CHAPTER 18

ONE DAY AT A TIME

DAILY

In one day Chippy, the parakeet, was sucked in, washed up and blown over. The reporter who wrote an article about the event said the problems began when Chippy's owner decided to clean Chippy's cage with a vacuum cleaner. Chippy's owner had removed the attachment from the end of the hose and stuck it in the cage; just then the phone rang and she turned to pick it up. Immediately Chippy got sucked into the vacuum. The bird owner gasped, put down the phone, turned off the vacuum and opened the bag and there was Chippy. He was still alive but he was stunned. Since the bird was covered with dust and soot (the article goes on to say), she grabbed him and raced him into the bathroom, turned on the tap and held Chippy under the water for ten minutes to get him clean, nearly drowning the bird. Then, realising that Chippy was soaked and shivering with cold, she did what any compassionate bird owner would do. She reached for the hair dryer and blew him dry for ten minutes. Poor Chippy didn't know what hit him. A few days after this drama, the reporter who had initially written about the event contacted Chippy's owner to see how the bird was recovering. "Well," she replied, 'Chippy doesn't sing much any more. He just kind of sits and stares into space."[41]

---

41 http://www.hopefulheart.net/thought-of-the-day/the-story-of-chippy

Have you ever felt sucked in, washed up and blown over by life? Life is tough and sometimes things hit you all at once so you begin to despair. It's called getting the hope kicked out of you.

Maybe you feel hopeless about a marriage situation and you think it's just not getting any better. Maybe you feel hopeless that you're never going to get married. Some may feel hopeless about whether they are ever going to have a child. Some feel hopeless about the child they have. You may feel hopeless about a financial situation or that the situation you're in is never going to change. Then there is the sense of hopelessness for the one with the ups and downs of bipolar disorder. Will this ever stabilise in my life? Will I ever be able to function normally again? Because certain situations have not gone our way, we assume that God was working against us. At times, we can become our own worst enemy. Because of relapses, failures and disappointments with recovery we can be filled with doubts, anxieties and phobias. We feel sucked in, washed up and blown over by bipolar.

If you have bipolar disorder, disappointments are going to happen to you, it's unavoidable. The question is how you choose to handle them. Are you going to obsess about them and get depressed? Are you going to let your failed expectations ruin your day? We must recognise that disappointments are a part of life, whether you have bipolar disorder or not.

Imagine you were feeling well and go out to dinner with friends. All of a sudden your mood changes and you don't want to be out anymore. You know you have to leave. You feel disappointed. You have the choice of berating yourself because your mood changed, blaming your bipolar disorder, picking a fight with your spouse (even blaming him), sulking, obsessing over it, getting depressed, or any number of other negative choices. Or you can just accept it as a disappointment, realising that they do happen. Readjust your focus and go on with your life.

If you are going to live with bipolar and try to manage the tensions between the highs and lows, you have to accept a lot of things simply because you have a mental illness. There is no shame in this. It's an attitude shift to accept the bipolar interruptions, because if you don't, they may very well become a trigger to the instability of your disorder.

One positive thing you can do with a disappointment, or any other unexpected change in your life, is to inject any kind of humour you can to diffuse the situation. It can't hurt and it can certainly help. *"A merry heart doeth good like a medicine: but a broken spirit drieth the bones." (Proverbs 17:22)*

One time in 2011 whilst Jenny was in hospital, I was studying the life of Noah in the Bible. I felt like Jenny's extended bipolar episode was like the forty days of rain that Noah and his family experienced. As the low episode continued with seemingly no change and no end in sight, I wondered how Noah felt on the ark not knowing if the rain would ever stop.

One day the rain did stop and the flooding stage was complete. Then began the next stage – floating. Noah and his family floated for 150 days. (Genesis 7:24-8:3) Have you ever escaped from a difficulty but the after effects continued? For 150 days there were 6 metres (20 feet) of water over the highest point on earth. Everything was covered with water. It took only 40 days to flood the earth but it took 150 days before the ark stopped floating and rested on land. Then it was another 150 days before all the water had dried up from off the earth. What the Lord taught me was that when you go through a trial, things don't go back to normal straight away. There is often a floating time. Just be patient. After the storm things don't look the same as they did before the storm. After a bipolar episode things don't look the same as they did prior to losing your mental health.

We live in the city of Rockhampton and have experienced several floods.[42] The Floods provide you with a different view afterward. It's always a different picture from what it was before the flood. Much has been altered and affected by the flood waters. As the danger of the flood waters subsides, then comes the 'floating' stage - the clean up and rebuilding. The recovery stage is always much longer than the flood itself.

We have found the same to be true with the 'flood' of any bipolar episode. The floating stage of recovery following a low or high moment can take weeks and even months. Floating time lasts much longer than the storm.

I wonder what Noah and his family thought during the 'floating' stage. The rain was gone but the trial was still continuing in another form. They didn't know when the ark would finally come to rest or when the water would abate. But God wasn't going to open the door until the coast was clear.

It's during the waiting times that we can become frustrated and tired of being couped up. Noah went from being a builder to being a vet. He went from walking in freedom to feeling trapped in the ark. No doubt he went from thinking he had all the answers, to having more questions.

Finally the ark came to rest upon the mountains of Ararat and stability began to return to Noah's life. After eight months had passed

---

42 The Fitzroy River catchment, due to its immense size and shape, is capable of producing severe flooding following heavy rainfall events. The Rockhampton Region has been affected by regular floods across recorded history. The latest major flooding from the Fitzroy River occurred in 1991, 2011 and again in 2013.

the mountain tops could be seen again. Noah then released a dove and a raven from the ark in a hope that they would return with a sign of vegetation or life. The raven never returned. The dove did return - but with nothing in its beak. After another week he released the dove again but this time the dove returned with an olive leaf in its beak, a sign that trees were emerging from the waters as they subsided. There was still more waiting time until Noah and his family were finally able to exit the ark. The total time in confinement before they left the ark was 370 days. The rains lasted forty days but there was a year of after effects.

What we see in Noah is patience and faithfulness to God. Noah stayed in the ark and even though it was a messy and stinky place, it was a safe place. You might be in a stinky place but God said you will come out of it. You might be in a stormy place but God said you will come out of it. You might be in a tight place but God said you will come out of it. You might be in an uncomfortable place but God said you will come out of it. Take one day at a time placing your faith in God. *"(For we walk by faith, not by sight:)"* (2 Corinthians 5:7)

Your bipolar effects may go on for a while after your episode, but readjust your focus and be patient, God has not forgotten you. A comforting section of scripture in this account says – *"And God remembered Noah..."* (Genesis 8:1)

Noah had no control over the past or the future, he couldn't change either. All Noah could do was live each day faithfully before God. I (Jenny) have learned, like Noah, to just take one day at a time. To live with concerns about yesterday and worries over the future is absolutely futile. I have no control over yesterday or tomorrow. Tomorrow isn't here yet and worrying about what might happen is only going to stress me out today. Again, there is absolutely nothing I can do about it and it will only make my bipolar disorder worse. The only day I have control over is today. So I have to make today count and make it the best day that I can. I have to take things as they come and live with my bipolar with this verse of scripture in mind: *"This is the day which the LORD hath made; we will rejoice and be glad in it."* *(Psalm 118:24)*

We all have daily challenges and having bipolar creates some more challenges of itself. The best way I have dealt with these is to stay in the moment and not to think too far ahead. By not overreacting, by not carrying yesterday's garbage on our backs, or worrying about tomorrow before it's even here, or being overly concerned about what other people think about us... we have a better chance of facing what is in front of us.

I (Jenny) have found that seeking to manage my bipolar and the problems that inevitably come with it one day at a time has been the most effective method for me. To start thinking too far ahead and guessing how long the episode will last, only seems to add additional pressure and stress to my life. My goal is to lean on God's grace day by day rather than thinking week by week or month by month.

The Bible speaks about the need to live day by day. *"For which cause we faint not; but though our outward man perish, yet the inward man is renewed day by day."* *(2 Corinthians 4:16)*

We must learn to live day by day and trust God for each day and not get too far ahead of ourselves. We look at a block of time and wonder, how we will cope for two months in hospital? The answer is not to look at the whole period of time but rather learn to live one day at a time without stressing over the future. If you keep thinking about the two months or the six weeks, it can become overwhelming and discouraging.

Someone once asked, "How do you read the Bible faithfully for the rest of your life?" The answer is by reading it one day at a time. When you finish one day, you then begin the next day and are faithful to God that day. Don't worry and wonder if you will be able to read the Bible every day for the whole year, just be faithful today. Begin today and then end today being faithful to God.

When the Lord Jesus was giving His disciples a pattern for prayer he taught them to pray, *"Give us this day our daily bread" (Matthew 6:11).* In Luke's gospel account the Lord taught them on another occasion a similar prayer, *"Give us day by day our daily bread." (Luke 11:3)*

In a day when our pantry cupboards are stocked and our refrigerators are full, why would we need to pray for more daily bread? We are living in a generation where many are eating too much bread. Some might ask, "Why would we pray for more?" It is a seemingly unnecessary prayer in this day and age. Many are fighting the battle of the bulge and are losing this battle. But the issue is not just bread. The issue is about total dependence on God every day.

The issue is learning to pray requests to God, acknowledging He is the all powerful provider. In the twenty first century in Australia, bread is not much of a daily need, but there are other needs God can meet. Some have an emotional need that really is a day to day issue. Others are in a marriage relationship and the issue is not whether you will have food tomorrow; the issue is, "Can I trust God to keep my marriage together today?" Our daily need for God is still just as great as it has always been throughout history.

It reminds me of a prayer I read a while back: "Dear Lord, so far today I'm doing all right. I've not gossiped, lost my temper, been greedy, grumpy, nasty, selfish or self indulgent. I've not lied, complained, cursed, or eaten any chocolate. I've not given in to temptation and used my credit card once today. But I'll be getting out of bed in a minute and I think I'm going to need Your help."[43]

God is the great provider of ALL our daily needs. We need to live in a DAY by DAY relationship with God especially in both the high and low bipolar episodes.

Coming back to our illustration and lesson from the life of Noah, we need to simply rely on and trust the Lord in the day by day 'floating' days. There will be times in life when we know some things for sure and other times we just don't know what is happening or where we will end up. It is during these day by day floating times when we have to learn to live in the 'in between' moments. The apostle Paul spoke about times like this where we must call on God to help us in the *"we know not"* stage of life. He mentions there are things *"we know"* in verses 22 and 28, but in between what we do know there are things *"we know not"* in verse 26.

*"**For we know** that the whole creation groaneth and travaileth in pain together until now."(Romans 8:22) … "Likewise the Spirit also helpeth our infirmities: **for we know not** what we should pray for as we ought: but the Spirit itself maketh intercession for us with groanings which cannot be uttered." (Romans 8:26) … "**And we know** that all things work together for good to them that love God, to them who are the called according to his purpose."(Romans 8:28)*

It's the 'in between' times we need to trust God day by day. It is in the middle that we have uncertainty. Do I have what it takes? Can I really get through this? We must replace self dependency with God's ability.

Lina Sandell of Sweden was the daughter of a pastor and being a frail youngster, she usually preferred to spend her time in her

43 http://iheartinspiration.com/quotes/dear-lord-so-far-today-i-have-not/

father's study rather than to join her friends in play. She became a hymn writer and when she was 26 years of age, she accompanied her father on a journey to Gothenburg, but tragedy occurred before the destination was reached. The ship gave a sudden lurch and Lina's father fell overboard and drowned before the eyes of his devoted daughter. She penned this hymn that flowed out of her broken heart.

Day by day, and with each passing moment,
Strength I find to meet my trials here;
Trusting in my Father's wise bestowment,
I've no cause for worry or for fear.
He, whose heart is kind beyond all measure,
Gives unto each day what He deems best,
Lovingly its part of pain and pleasure,
Mingling toil with peace and rest.
Every day the Lord Himself is near me,
With a special mercy for each hour;
All my cares He fain would bear and cheer me,
He whose name is Counsellor and Pow'r.
The protection of His child and treasure
Is a charge that on Himself He laid;
"As thy days, thy strength shall be in measure,"
This the pledge to me He made.
Help me then, in every tribulation,
So to trust Thy promises, O Lord,
That I lose not faith's sweet consolation,
Offered me within Thy holy Word.
Help me, Lord, when toil and trouble meeting,
E'er to take, as from a father's hand,
One by one, the days, the moments fleeting,
Till with Christ the Lord I stand.

PART 3

THERAPIES TO LEARN

CHAPTER 19

25 PRACTICAL SOLUTIONS

DOING

On 17th of August 2015 I (Jenny) completed a ten week course on learning strategies to better control mood swings that occur with my bipolar disorder. Even though I have lived with this mental illness for twenty-three years at the time of writing this book, I am still learning new ways to help manage my life. I have learned that bipolar involves cycling moods, which are accompanied by a wide range of other symptoms that affect not just mood but also energy, memory, thinking and interaction with other people. I have been constantly developing my 'bipolar toolbox' to help control my mood swings. By combining some of the available treatments I can achieve a good management plan that aids in maintaining my well-being and limiting the cycle of recurring depression and mania.

We believe that mental illness is very complex and so it must be addressed by each individual at multiple levels. If you're going to get well, if you're going to stay healthy, if you're going to help others maintain their mental well-being, you're going to have to deal with the physical, social, emotional, mental and spiritual levels. The most basic level is the physical part of our lives. It involves the brain chemistry, good overall health, diet, exercise and getting enough sleep. These are biological factors affecting your mental health. The more complicated levels of our life are the social, emotional, mental and spiritual areas. This involves learning healthy ways of managing our mind and thoughts. We believe the Bible has a lot to say about managing our moods by managing the way we think. You cannot control every thought that comes in to your mind, but you can control what you choose to do with it and where you choose to get help.

As a couple, we have found there are some general forms of treatment and therapies that are available to anyone who lives with bipolar and then there are some other specific spiritual practices that offer additional help to a Christian. It's with this premise in mind that we humbly offer the following suggestions for those living with bipolar disorder.

PART 1 – GENERAL TREATMENT AND THERAPIES

Prescriptions - Medications

The key with any severe mental illness is appropriate medications and as we said previously, brain science is not an exact science. Everyone must be individually prescribed with medicine that is right for them. In fact, one person's medicine may very well be another person's poison. There is no one tablet that suits all patients with a mental illness.

It has been proven that the symptoms of depression, mania, mood swings, anxiety, irritability and bad sleep patterns can be effectively controlled with or without medication. However, mood disorders such as bipolar are a biological illness that causes changes in the way your brain processes the chemicals your body naturally produces; therefore if you choose not to take medication you will limit a source of treatment that is definitely effective for people who have severe mood swings. Denial of the need to use medication is something I (Jenny) have experienced. Early in my prognosis, during a period of wellness, I hated taking my medication so I decided to stop taking them. Five weeks later I ended up in a major depressive state. From that experience I have now learned to listen to the advice of my doctors. Consistent use of prescribed medications, acceptance of the illness and the right mix of medication will help you to live a normal life.

Don't forget to take your medication, wherever you are. If you're going to be somewhere other than at home when it's time to take your medication, be sure you have it with you. Pillboxes are good for this. Plan ahead of time. If you do happen to miss a dose (we're all human), just make sure you take the next dose. If you are travelling overseas, see your doctor beforehand and take a letter from him/her listing all your medication. Also take extra prescriptions with you in case you run out of a medication whilst you are away. It is very difficult to get a doctor who does not know you to prescribe psychiatric medication based on your request. Once while travelling to the United States of America, I forgot a certain medication and had no back-up prescriptions with me. It took us almost an entire day to find a doctor and explain my situation enough and prove I needed the medication! I'm still learning much about my illness and keep in close contact with my caring and wonderful general practitioner, Dr Sandy Prasad and my lovely psychiatrist, Dr Lynne Steele, to keep my medication and lifestyle in check, so as to live a normal lifestyle.

Psychotherapy – *Psychologists, Psychiatrists, Therapists, Counsellors*

We believe psychotherapy is an essential complement to medical treatment for people with bipolar disorder. There is a need for both medical and psychological 'tools' to encourage bipolar sufferers to become more than passive pill takers and learn new coping skills. Professional counselling helps patients deal with the emotional problems and stresses that trigger the onset of manic or depressive episodes. It can also resolve many of the unstable relational problems, internal struggles and depressive moods that accompany acute phases of the disorder. Medication alone does not have nearly such a positive effect as medication combined with good, long-term, ongoing psychotherapy. Secular psychiatrists and psychologists operate on a biopsychosocial model of human development and behaviour. The belief and use of scripture and the Gospel is perhaps the most prevalent difference between the secular and Christian psychology worlds. The secular model proposes that humans develop and operate only according to biological, psychological and social influences. Accordingly, we are products of our biology and environment, both bearing equal importance. In more recent years, psychologists have begun recognizing that our spirituality impacts our lives, but have yet to say it is imperative for life. While the traditional psychological theories and models that are based upon naturalism are insufficient from a Christian worldview, not all of secular psychology is wrong. Indeed, there are many helpful and positive aspects of psychology to consider. For instance, learning about the intricacies of the human brain, the environmental influences on our personality and the social and cultural impact on our lives does help in developing coping strategies to aid in avoiding relapses. We believe the use of some secular therapy and interventions are extremely helpful, with research and personal testimonies revealing their success in the abatement of symptoms. Helping people organise their time, challenging negative thoughts, teaching diaphragmatic breathing and providing life-skill training that may help alleviate their psychological distress, are all helpful and needful secular techniques.

Practical life skills

These are gained in psychotherapy or in educational groups led by trained teachers. I (Jenny) have been able to glean much from some of the workshop sessions I have been involved with during times of hospitalisation. Classes that help strengthen stress management skills and healthy habits will also help avoid mood swings. There are many skills that can be learned and enhanced to build confidence in life. These include practical things like interviewing for a job, finding housing and making friends. Psychological things include receiving comfort in grief, assertiveness training, moderating moods and using positive self-talk. Even learning to laugh at life is a skill to be learned. As critical as medications are, using pills alone can't keep you at optimum stability. No drug can teach you how to get along with someone, have a stress-free job interview, handle criticism, or overcome disappointment. To heal, recover and rebuild successfully will take more than meds. You will need more people to lean on and workable strategies, techniques and practical life skills.

Perception of triggers

Research suggests that most mind illnesses are caused by a combination of genetic and environmental factors that interact with each other in complex ways. This means that stress, successes, relationships, attitudes, habits and other factors may at times be triggers that influence initial and subsequent episodes of a mental illness like bipolar disorder. When someone starts to 'fly' into a manic episode or 'slide' into a depressive episode or 'break' into a psychotic episode, it needs to be nipped in the bud. These episodes can be damaging to the person's psyche. The quicker the treatment is administered the better. We urge people to seek help immediately when they start to notice signs of an episode. Relationship breakups, the loss of a loved one, sleep changes, becoming sentimental about events and anniversaries, stress and seasons of the year can be triggers for many people with bipolar disorder. For me the main trigger is lack of routine sleep. I need at least eight hours of sleep each night. I also learned that I have sleep apnoea. With a medical test done over night in hospital it was determined that I needed a CPAP (Continuous Positive Airways Pressure) machine to enable me to get a sound sleep at night. This helps me immensely to stay healthy. Also, Christmas is that time of the year that can be very exciting. It can be too easy to fall prey to a manic or depressive episode if I'm not careful. Learn to monitor and track your mood swings and begin to recognise any changes in your mood. Some people use mood charts to record their daily moods. I (Jenny) use a diary system and write daily notes about my mood and events that have happened. I have learnt to use my diary as a tool to help monitor my mood and also show my doctor and psychiatrist how I'm going. The more information and description of my symptoms makes it easier for my doctor and psychiatrist to provide appropriate medication for me and a plan to cope with the onset of my mood swing. Usually, after Christmas each year I will go back over my diary and rejoice over how much the Lord has helped me accomplish that year.

Pattern of Sleep

Monitor your sleep habits. Bipolar disorder is closely tied to a person's core body rhythms, so stick to a regular sleep schedule. Losing sleep could lead to an episode if you're not careful. Excessive social gatherings may disrupt your sleep patterns, so be sure to watch your sleep habits carefully. During and coming out of a particularly low episode all I (Jenny) want to do is curl up in bed, talk to nobody, be left alone and sleep the day away. Even though I feel this way I have learned not to listen to or give in to these feelings otherwise, I end up with my sleep routine all out of alignment resulting in either insomnia or at times hypersomnia. In an account in the Bible where the prophet Elijah was depressed and suicidal, God prescribed sleep. *"And as he lay and **slept** under a juniper tree, behold, then an angel touched him, and said unto him, Arise and eat. And he looked, and, behold, there was a cake baken on the coals, and a cruse of water at his head. And he did eat and drink, and **laid him down again**."* (1 Kings 19:5-6) Sometimes the most spiritual thing that you can do is rest.

Proper Nutrition – Eating

Eating a healthy diet and drinking plenty of water is part of managing your bipolar disorder. Nutritious foods are the best source of vitamins and minerals. I try to fill up with food from the vegetable and fruit food groups first, before eating the more fattening things. I have learned that having healthy eating helps manage my bipolar. One of the side effects of some medication is an increased appetite, especially after the evening meal. I have found drinking water and having prepared low sugar and low fat snacks has helped to alleviate cravings. Minimise caffeine intake and abstain from the use of nonprescribed drugs or alcohol. Stimulants can trigger a depressed bipolar person to flip into a manic episode, while sedatives can trigger a depressive phase.

Physical exercise

Stick to an exercise routine. Walking is one of the best forms of exercise. We have a highly energetic dog named "Jack", an Australian Terrier, which I take for a walk a few times a week. Actually he takes me for a walk. I have found when I do regular exercise it helps my mind think more clearly. A simple thing you can do when you go to the shopping mall, is park farther away from the shops so that you have a longer walk to the door. I have also found doing water aerobics twice a week has helped my physical stamina and mental state.

Planning

Certain times of the year will be more exacting than at others. For example Christmas time is often very exciting involving a lot of activities. There are parties, lots of people you haven't seen since last year and exchanging of gifts. Make sure you don't let your excitement get out of hand. Don't make more preparations than you can handle. Don't overdo things, just pace yourself. Instead of the pressure of doing that last-minute shopping and the noise and hassle of the crowded shopping malls, plan to do your Christmas shopping ahead of time. Make a list and stick to it. It will make your shopping easier and be less stressful for you. Holidays don't have to be a trigger for an episode. Stick as closely to your normal routines as possible.

This will help you manage your bipolar and make it through the holidays okay.

Pay for help

We employ a house cleaner for one hour a week to help vacuum, mop, clean the bathroom and general tidying up. The reason we budget to provide for this from week to week is we never know when I (Jenny) will be unwell. This way we can be sure the basic necessities are taken care of and kept clean. I am very thankful to the wonderful ladies who have assisted me over the years. They have been such a blessing to our family.

Pull Away from Stress

Sometimes being around large noisy crowds and even being around family can be very stressful for someone with bipolar disorder. Try to avoid the critical attitudes from family and friends. If one of your family members' complaining gets on your nerves and is causing you stress, ease away from them at the first chance you get. If the noise from all the children makes you stressed, try to stay in another part of the house. If it will help you feel better, don't attend the family gathering this year – just tell them that you're not up to it. They'll usually understand.

Physicians – *Doctors*

Keep your regular appointments with your doctor/psychiatrist, even when you are feeling well and during holiday times. Make sure, however, that you check with them in advance about their holiday schedule as they may take this time to be with their own families. Also check if they have emergency plans in case you need them during this time and the offices are closed, or you run out of medication.

People in your life – *Support from family and friends*

Discuss with family members ahead of time a plan of action. It helps to deal with future episodes ahead of time. This is done most effectively when the bipolar person's insight and judgment are not impaired during the middle of an acute manic or depressive episode. When I am unwell I lean heavily on my husband, Robert, my boys Tim and JJ and friends from church. They work together to keep the household going until I'm better. Last time I was hospitalised I was away for three weeks and then it took another two weeks at home before I was functioning normally again. Build a support network to help you during the down moments. We have to learn to rely on the safety net of support, and to build safe people into our lives to fill our lives with the love and grace of others who walk with us.

Pleasures – *Hobbies and fun things*

Get out of the house and do things you enjoy. I love to work in my vegetable garden when I'm well and will aim to spend up to three hours a week out in the sunshine picking, planting and tending to the garden. I find this task very therapeutic. Sometimes I will go window

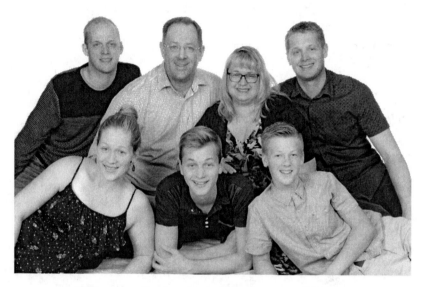

Back row – Benjamin, Robert, Jenny and Joshua.
Front row – Anna, Timothy and Jonathan (JJ)

shopping just for the exercise and enjoyment. I joined a local card-making group where I meet with other ladies once a week for two hours to be taught how to make beautiful personal cards. I have used cards I've made to be an encouragement to others who are ill or in need.

Projects – Small tasks

When feeling overwhelmed it is tempting to give up and lie in bed doing nothing. If I pick one task each day; break it down, pick a time to start and complete the task, then the feeling of accomplishing something is great. This is not always easy, but when you are low it can be obtainable. A routine works well for me whether I am balanced or unhealthy. I strive to rise at the same time every day, have breakfast and take my medication. It is important to take your meds at the same time every day if possible. I get dressed and do my daily devotions and write in my diary.

Printed material – Books and resources

Education on bipolar disorder is very helpful. Over the years we have read numerous books, articles, blogs and watched movies and documentaries on the issue. We have both attended mental health seminars and workshops. Some of the books we have found very useful include:

- *Broken Minds* by Steve & Robyn Bloem
- *Hope Again* by Mark Sutton and Bruce Hennigan
- *The Bipolar Disorder Survival Guide* by David J. Miklowitz
- *Hope, Help and Healing for the Depressed* by Mark Tossell
- *Grace for the Afflicted* by Matthew S. Stanford
- *Bipolar Disorder: Rebuilding your life* by Rev. Dr James T. Stout
- *Mental Health First Aid Manual* by Betty Kitchener, Anthony Jorm & Claire Kelly
- *Break the Bipolar Cycle* by Elizabeth Brondolo and Xavier Amador
- *The Bipolar Workbook* by Monica Ramirez Basco
- *The Bible Cure for Depression and Anxiety* by Don Colbert, M.D.

- *The Best of Times, The Worst of Times* by Penelope Rowe and Jessica Rowe

- *Coming out of the Dark* by Mary Southerland

- *Anxiety, Fear, And Depression* by Robert S. Peterson

Programs – Support groups

Join a support group in your local community, if it is available, that is specific to bipolar disorder. A support group with other individuals with bipolar disorder along with their family members can be a source of additional help. Since people with bipolar disorder often feel that no one understands their mood swings and erratic behaviour, support from others who have had similar experiences can be very helpful. At our church we have a program called 'Anchor' which offers a bipolar and mental health support group.

PART 2 – SPIRITUAL TREATMENT AND THERAPIES

Prayer

Prayer is powerful and prayer works. One of the great benefits of being a Christian is knowing you can talk to your Creator anytime, anywhere and about anything. Prayer is a means by which you can unload your concerns and cares upon a God who truly loves you and is interested in every detail of your life. While on earth the Lord Jesus prayed to the heavenly Father on many occasions, teaching us valuable principles on prayer. The Bible is full of examples of answered prayer and people who prayed. As a couple we have the opportunity to pray together to God during the crisis moments in bipolar episodes. This provides us with so much comfort knowing we have a God who hears us and answers prayer.

Places of worship - *Church*

Whilst on earth, Jesus came back to Nazareth, the place where he grew up and went into the local synagogue. He took the scroll of Isaiah, unrolled it to a certain passage and began reading. The account is as follows: *"And he came to Nazareth, where he had been brought up: and, as his custom was, he went into the synagogue on the sabbath day, and stood up for to read. And there was delivered unto him the book of the prophet Esaias. And when he had opened the book, he found the place where it was written, The Spirit of the Lord is upon me, because he hath anointed me to preach the gospel to the poor; he hath sent me to heal the brokenhearted, to preach deliverance to the captives, and recovering of sight to the blind, to set at liberty them that are bruised, To preach the acceptable year of the Lord. And he closed the book, and he gave it again to the minister, and sat down. And the eyes of all them that were in the synagogue were fastened on him. And he began to say unto them, This day is this scripture fulfilled in your ears."* (Luke 4:16-21) Jesus was saying that He was the Messiah referred to in Isaiah and was going to fulfil the prophecies. In essence He said, "I'm going to stand with those who suffer." Today God has given the local church the same mission to stand with people who suffer. Some of the people who suffer the greatest in our society, in our world, are people living with mental illness. This is why places of worship are so helpful for people living with bipolar. The church has a unique opportunity to do something that nobody else can do. It can step up and care for people in ways that nobody else can, to care and have compassion. Churches provide much needed Christian fellowship and help people learn to accept and face their suffering as part of living in a fallen, sinful world.

They can also help people have lasting hope that the best of life is yet to come: life in eternity with our Heavenly Father. Faith, in other words, can help people live well with their disorder. Admittedly not all churches are equipped or sympathetic towards those living with a mental illness, but that is by no means a reflection on God. Some churches do fail to provide adequate help because they think they can give simple religious platitudes for a complex matter. If you haven't found a church that can assist you in your journey with bipolar, keep looking. They do exist. Sometimes showing up at church is incredibly hard, but if you just show up, God will be there, ministry will be there and the community will be there. Nobody can offer hope like Jesus. The government can't offer much hope. Professionals can offer some hope with medication and therapy. But the church can offer the hope of Jesus that sustains you in your darkest days.

Patience – Waiting on God

Learning the theological truths of the nature and work of God enables you to understand better the plans and purposes of God. Reading the stories and accounts of the Bible where people waited on God to speak, move, deliver, judge and work provides the reader with principles for their own life. Knowing God makes all the difference in learning to wait patiently on Him. *"Wait on the LORD: be of good courage, and he shall strengthen thine heart: wait, I say, on the LORD."* *(Psalm 27:14)*

Praise – *Singing to and about God*

Listening to godly Christian music and praising the Lord in song strengthens your heart and mind. Music actually teaches us and reaffirms the truths we believe – *"Let the word of Christ dwell in you richly in all wisdom; teaching and admonishing one another in psalms and hymns and spiritual songs, singing with grace in your hearts to the Lord."* *(Colossians 3:16)* Music has been a great source of therapy for the soul and mind.

Promises – *God's Word*

The promises of God are sure and never fail. There are over seven thousand promises in God's Word that Christians can claim. The promises connected to peace, joy and fear are of tremendous benefit to the person suffering with bipolar. To know and read the promises of God and trust in them provides much needed stability and clarity of mind. I (Jenny) have found reading my Bible becomes a source of inspiration, encouragement and motivation. I read as much or as little as I can consume with my mind each day. Some days that means one verse of scripture, other days I can read a few chapters. I also read a book full of scriptures called "Daily Light."[44] I have found this book to be very refreshing and timely in my life as I read the daily passages. One of the greatest promises in the Word of God is that what isn't healed on earth will be in Heaven. *"And God shall wipe away all tears from their eyes; and there shall be no more death, neither sorrow, nor crying, neither shall there be any more pain: for the former things are passed away."* *(Revelation 21:4)* You can also obtain a *Bible*

---

44 An online version of *Daily Light* can be found at http://www.dailylightdevotional. org/

Promise Book[45] that contains the promises in the Bible arranged in topics. This is a good resource and easy to use.

Pondering – Meditation on God's works, world and Word

Bible meditation is recommended for the Christian as a practice to stimulate your thoughts and memory. As you go through life it is important to maintain a biblical world view of what is happening in and around you and think upon what God is doing. Look for the Lord's hand and ways in His world, works and Word. *"I will remember the works of the LORD: surely I will remember thy wonders of old. I will meditate also of all thy work, and talk of thy doings." (Psalm 77:11-12)* Thinking upon the Lord and His workings will help you keep a right perspective on life.

Preaching – Sermons from the Word of God

Sitting under the preaching and teaching of God's Word provides you with a steady diet of spiritual food to nourish your heart, soul and mind. We have both found over the years that the topics and passages of scripture being expounded are exactly what we needed to hear for where we were at in our lives. Without a doubt the pulpit ministry of the church provides much needed direction and guidance in a world that has its values contrary to the Word of God.

---

45 A Kindle version is available at https://www.amazon.com/Bible-Promise-Book-KJV-ebook/dp/B002WIG3S6

Pastor – *Having a shepherd to talk to*

We know that pastors and police are often the first responders in a mental health crisis. Having the ability to talk with a trusted pastor who cares for you is a blessing. The Bible likens us to sheep that need nurturing, feeding and guiding. God in His wisdom gives pastors and teachers to the body of Christ and gifts them to do the work they do for Him. Whilst I (Robert) am a pastor, I have also benefited from pastoral counsel in my life. "*Where no counsel is, the people fall: but in the multitude of counsellors there is safety.*" *(Proverbs 11:14)* As a pastor I counsel people who may struggle with a mental illness that their illness is not their identity. If they are a follower of Jesus Christ then their identity is in Him. Their primary identity is in their Creator and Saviour.

Personal relationship with God – *Being born again*

The great spiritual therapy and treatment that any person can have is to be born again. Jesus said, "*... Verily, verily, I say unto thee, Except a man be born again, he cannot see the kingdom of God. ...Marvel not that I said unto thee, Ye must be born again.*" *(John 3:3,7)* If you have never trusted Christ as your personal Saviour and been born again, may I invite you to consider four simple truths to guide you to redemption.

All have sinned against God

First, the Bible says, *"For all have sinned, and come short of the glory of God..."* (Romans 3:23) You may have heard someone say, "I'm only human - nobody's perfect." This Bible verse says the same thing: We are all sinners. We all do things that we know are wrong. We have broken the laws of God and that's why we feel separated from God - because God is holy and we are not. The Bible says, *"Wherefore, as by one man sin entered into the world, and death by sin; and so death passed upon all men, for that all have sinned..."* (Romans 5:12)

Sin must be punished by God

Just as criminals must pay the penalty for their crimes, the Bible says that sinners must pay the penalty for their sins. If you continue to sin, you will pay the penalty of spiritual death. *"For the wages of sin is death; but the gift of God is eternal life through Jesus Christ our Lord."* (Romans 6:23) Somebody has to pay for all the things you've ever done wrong – either you or somebody else. Either you go to hell or somebody else pays for all the things you've done wrong. That's what justice demands. You will not only die physically; you will also be separated from our holy God for all eternity. The Bible teaches that those who choose to remain separated from God will spend eternity in a place called hell. *"And death and hell were cast into the lake of fire. This is the second death. And whosoever was not found written in the book of life was cast into the lake of fire." (Revelation 20:14-15)*

The Lord Jesus Christ paid the penalty for your sin

Jesus Christ came to Earth, lived a perfect life and died on the cross for your sins. It's all been paid for - every sin you have ever committed - even the ones you haven't done yet. They've already been paid for. The Bible teaches that Jesus Christ, the sinless Son of God, paid the penalty for all your sins when He was crucified. You may think you have to lead a good life and do good deeds before God will love you. But the Bible says that Christ loved you enough to die for you, even when you were rebelling against Him. You must believe that the Lord Jesus Christ died on the cross and shed his blood for your sins, was buried and that God did raise him from the dead. The Bible says *"But God commendeth his love toward us, in that, while we were yet sinners, Christ died for us." (Romans 5:8)* It is through the shedding of Christ's blood we have forgiveness of sins. The Bible speaks of Christ and says *"In whom we have redemption through his blood, the forgiveness of sins, according to the riches of his grace" (Ephesians 1:7)* If there had been any other way for you to be saved from your sin so you could go to a heaven when you die, don't you think God would have chosen the less painful way? If there had been two ways to get to heaven, don't you think He would have used the other way rather than let His Son go through all that suffering? The fact is, friend, there is no other way. If there were any other way, Jesus Christ's death is a waste. The only way you have any chance of getting to heaven is accepting the free forgiveness of Jesus Christ who paid for it on the cross. That is the only way you'll ever get into heaven.

You must repent of your sin and personally accept Christ as your Saviour

Jesus Christ wants to have a personal relationship with you. Picture, if you will, Jesus Christ standing at the door of your heart knocking. Invite Him in; He is waiting for you to receive Him into your heart and life. Admit you're a sinner and need to be saved from Hell. Be willing to turn from your sins (repent). We must trust Jesus Christ as Lord and Saviour and receive Him by personal invitation *"For whosoever shall call upon the name of the Lord shall be saved." (Romans 10:13)* The Lord Jesus called this being 'born again.'

Are you willing to ask Jesus to be your Saviour? Then please ask Him to save your soul in a prayer like this:

"Dear Lord, I know I'm a sinner and if I died tonight I wouldn't go to heaven. I believe that Jesus Christ died on the cross in my place, shed His blood for my sin, was buried and rose again from the dead. With all my heart I turn from my sin and ask Jesus Christ to be my personal Saviour and come into my heart right now, forgive my sins, and take me to heaven when I die. Thank you Lord for saving me today, Amen."

If you just prayed and trusted Christ as your Saviour, you can be sure you are going to Heaven when you die. Congratulations!

CHAPTER 20

FREQUENTLY ASKED QUESTIONS

DISCUSSION

What causes bipolar disorder?

Physiological factors appear to play the most important role in causing bipolar disorder. There is some evidence of a genetic link. Emotional factors, however, such as excessive stress and loss of close relationships, can trigger the disorder.

Can a person be cured of bipolar?

With God all things are possible. If He chooses to heal a person of bipolar He can. People suffering from bipolar disorder and their family members can receive great strength from their faith in Christ as well as their dependence on the Word of God. From a human standpoint, there is no medical cure for bipolar illness; only the ability to manage the symptoms. Most sufferers, however, can remain relatively symptom-free if they comply rigidly with their medical regime, receive competent, ongoing counselling by a pastor or therapist who understands the issues of the disorder, and adjust their lifestyle to avoid known triggers.

Can a person with bipolar disorder keep his/her job?

This will depend on the severity of the illness for each person. Generally, people who are compliant with medications, continue psychotherapy and adjust their lifestyle are able to live well-balanced for most of their lives. If or when they do have recurrences, family understanding and proper medication can generally restabilise them in a relatively short period of time.

How often do people relapse?

Some people have patterns of illness that are more severe. They may relapse more frequently or their illness may be more resistant to treatment. On average most people have an episode every 2 to 3 years. However, some people with bipolar disorder remain well for many years and others relapse very frequently. People who relapse 4 or more times a year are considered to have rapid cycling. With time and treatment rapid cycling can change and the person may keep well for longer periods of time. Don't give up hope as patterns of illness can change.

Does bipolar illness involve demon possession?

No. Many committed Christians suffer from bipolar disorder and, like non-Christians, they respond to medications like lithium carbonate. When a person responds to medications, that is clear evidence that the problem is physical or emotional—not a matter of demon possession.

How can psychotherapy help?

Acceptance of the illness is a major step to recovery. Professional psychologists, psychiatrists and counsellors can help a person understand bipolar and accept themselves with their disorder. Illnesses such as bipolar disorder can tear at one's self-esteem and make one feel lonely, isolated and cut off from others. Through wise, effective biblical counselling a person can grow stronger emotionally and spiritually learning to manage their moods and handle the conflicts and stresses that can sometimes arise in an acute phase of the disorder. Psychotherapy can also assist patients and their families to deal with family struggles better and to work together to deal with any episodes.

Who would be a wise counsellor for me?

As a Christian, the first place to go is to your pastor. If he is not equipped to deal with the unique challenges of bipolar you may need to also look for a Christian psychologist who has helped others with the disorder. If you can't immediately find a wise group of counsellors, remember that wisdom is rooted in the fear of the Lord. So look for someone who has a growing knowledge of Jesus Christ and a track record of spiritual faithfulness. Investigate bipolar disorder together with such a person.

Are there any side effects of the medical treatments for bipolar disorder?

Yes, there often are. But the consequences of not taking medication may be worse. It is highly advisable to continue under your medical treatment as prescribed. Avoid self-diagnosing and self-medicating. If you have any medication or medical questions or concerns always consult with your doctor.

How long does it take for medication to work?

Often within one to two weeks of commencing treatment. Some medications such as Lithium may take longer to find precisely the correct dosage within the therapeutic range. The correct dosage is the one that provides optimal relief of symptoms with a minimum of side effects.

What about antidepressants? Where did they come from?

During the 1950s, researchers trying to develop a cure for tuberculosis discovered a class of medication that had no effect on the infection but elevated the mood of ill, depressed patients. By accident, the first antidepressants were developed.

Are mood stabilizers different from antidepressants?

Mood stabilizers are used to control mood swings among patients with bipolar disorder. They act by decreasing the activity of the brain to restore neurochemical balance. They are given to treat positive and negative symptoms of bipolar mood disorder. Lithium is the prototype of mood stabilizers and is the universally preferred treatment of bipolar mood disorder. Anticonvulsant medications such as Valproate, whilst originally designed for treating epilepsy, have been found to also be useful in controlling unstable moods by decreasing the rate of neuronal firing necessary for brain activity. On the other hand, antidepressant medications work by preventing the breakdown of the neurotransmitters that allow the spark to jump from one nerve cell to another across the synapse. The medication essentially increases the levels of such chemicals as serotonin which is necessary for proper function of nerves. They are given to patients with depressive symptoms and disorders such as major depression, seasonal affective disorder, psychotic depression and depressive phase of bipolar mood disorder.

Are there side effects to anti-depressant medication?

In general, anti-depressant medications produce a host of similar side effects. These can include blurred vision, dry mouth, changes in sexual function, sleep disruption, drowsiness and appetite changes. However, not all of these drugs produce all of these side effects. This is why it is so important to allow your doctor or psychiatrist to tailor the medication to your specific needs. Some side effects go away with time.

Can you get addicted to antidepressants?

Antidepressants are not addictive. Think of your medication as a diabetic thinks of insulin. You need it to function.

My family is terrified that I will be manic again. How can I help them?

It is important that you continue to listen to your family's fears. Encourage them to speak openly with you. Try to help them understand more about the disorder and ask them to help by spotting changes within your mood. Let them know your management plan for your mental well-being. Don't let shame or embarrassment prevent you from asking for help. Let your pastor know what is happening and invite him to help your family.

I am concerned about a loved one's mental health. How should I talk with him or her about it?

Prepare for the conversation, set the stage and create an inviting atmosphere. Discuss your concerns about your loved one's mental health when the person feels safe and comfortable; timing is everything. Communicate your observations in a straightforward manner and watch for reactions during the discussion and slow down or back up if the person becomes confused or looks upset. Ask questions like; "I have noticed you have seemed different lately (irritated, sad, distant, that you have a lot on your mind, distracted, distressed)." Or "I am concerned about you. How can I help?", "Can you tell me more about what is happening in your life (work, school, family, friends, home)?"; "Would you be open to talking with someone else (an adult, a pastor, a doctor, a therapist) about what's going on?"

How can I help a family member with bipolar disorder?

Pray that God will help him find a way of healing and help for him. Get professional help for that person as soon as you see a manic or depressive episode coming on. Help him comply with medical treatment. Be patient and encourage that person to accept himself with the disorder. If your family member becomes suicidal or a danger to himself or others, get help immediately from the police.

What tips can help family members cope when a loved one is diagnosed with bipolar disorder?

Many families who have a loved one with a mental illness may find themselves denying the warning signs, worrying what other people will think because of the stigma, or wondering what caused your loved one to become ill. It is not uncommon to question your faith, feel anger toward God and ask "Why?" Accept that these feelings are normal and common among families going through similar situations. Find out all you can about bipolar disorder by reading and talking with mental health professionals. Therapy can be beneficial for both the individual with a mental illness and other family members. A mental health professional can suggest ways to cope and better understand your loved one's illness.

How do I explain what bipolar disorder is to my child?

Young children need less information and fewer details because of a limited ability to understand. Preschool children focus primarily on things they can see. For example, they may have questions about a person who has an unusual physical appearance, or is behaving strangely. They would also be very aware of people who are crying and obviously sad, upset, or angry. Older children and teenagers may want more specifics. They may ask more questions, especially about friends or family with emotional or behavioural problems. It is important to answer their questions directly and honestly and to reassure them about their concerns and feelings. It is important to talk with your children and loved ones about their emotions.

How do I talk with someone who is suicidal?

If you suspect someone you know is suicidal, tell that person that you are worried and want to help. Don't be afraid to use the word "suicide." By simply asking, you will not put the idea in his mind. Ask whether he is considering taking his life and ask if he has a specific plan. Having a plan may indicate that he is farther along and needs help right away. Your direct, non-judgmental questions can encourage him to share his thoughts and feelings. Make sure the person knows you are in this moment together, you're with him and that he is loved and valued. Be genuine, caring and show respect; have a caring conversation. Don't lie or make promises you can't keep. Find something to refer to that the person can hope in: an upcoming event or their children or family. It is essential to help him find immediate professional care. If he tells you he is going to commit suicide, you must act immediately. Don't leave the person alone and don't try to argue. Instead, ask questions like, "Have you thought about how you'd do it?"; "Do you have the means?" and "Have you decided when you'll do it?" If the person has a defined plan - the means are easily available, the method is a lethal one and the time is set - then risk of suicide is obviously severe. In such an instance, the person needs to get to the nearest hospital emergency room. If you are together in person or talking on the phone together, you may even need to call the emergency number (000 in Australia, 911 in USA). Remember, under such circumstances no actions on your part should be considered too extreme—you are trying to save a life.

What should happen when you leave hospital?

Before leaving the hospital, individuals need to have a discharge plan. Make sure they have a written list of what medications to take, what dosage is required and when to take them. It is important to know that individuals might not feel better immediately. They should allow themselves to slowly and gradually get back to routine and to stick with their treatment plans. People leaving the hospital after surgery or another medical emergency need time for healing and recovery. It is no different for people leaving a hospital due to bipolar disorder treatment. People leaving the hospital are vulnerable and a gentle approach to reintegrating with the world can be helpful. It is important to know a person is not 'fixed' when leaving the hospital. It is likely the beginning of a longer-term recovery process. It is unrealistic to think a person can go back to his normal life right away. Don't be afraid to ask about how someone is doing and assure the person of your commitment to the relationship. Ask the person if you can help with practical needs and spend time together doing things like going to the park, playing a game or watching a movie.

A FINAL NOTE

For those who suffer with bipolar, whether you wake up as either Tigger or Eeyore, we pray that this book has provided you with some tools and encouragement to help you find hope when you are poles apart.

We pray that all our readers have a new empathetic understanding of the daily challenges faced by those who are afflicted with bipolar disorder or any other mental illness.

There are no cookie-cutter set answers that will be effective in every situation for this complex illness. We know first-hand there will be the bright days and the dark days and the best closing advice we can give you is in the words of King George VI when he gave his Christmas address to the British Empire in 1939 as they were plunged into the uncertainty of war. As part of this speech he quoted from Minnie Haskins' poem "The Gate of the Year" (1908):

> I said to the man who stood at the Gate of the Year, 'Give me a light that I may tread safely into the unknown.' And he replied, 'Go out into the darkness, and put your hand into the Hand of God. That shall be better than light, and safer than a known way.'

We know that our journey with bipolar will continue but we also know Who is walking with us – Jesus!

"For thou wilt light my candle: the LORD my God will enlighten my darkness." (Psalm 18:28)

SCRIPTURES FOR ENCOURAGEMENT

When you need hope

> **Romans 15:13** "Now the God of hope fill you with all joy and peace in believing, that ye may abound in hope, through the power of the Holy Ghost."

When you need sleep

> **Psalm 3:3-5** "But thou, O LORD, art a shield for me; my glory, and the lifter up of mine head. I cried unto the LORD with my voice, and he heard me out of his holy hill. Selah. I laid me down and slept; I awaked; for the LORD sustained me. But you, O LORD, are a shield about me, my glory, and the lifter of my head."

> **Psalm 4:8** "I will both lay me down in peace, and sleep: for thou, LORD, only makest me dwell in safety."

When you need refuge

> **Psalm 62:6-8** "He only is my rock and my salvation: he is my defence; I shall not be moved. In God is my salvation and my glory: the rock of my strength, and my refuge, is in

God. Trust in him at all times; ye people, pour out your heart before him: God is a refuge for us. Selah."

When you need strength

Psalm 73:26 "My flesh and my heart faileth: but God is the strength of my heart, and my portion for ever."

Isaiah 40:28-31 "Hast thou not known? hast thou not heard, that the everlasting God, the LORD, the Creator of the ends of the earth, fainteth not, neither is weary? there is no searching of his understanding. He giveth power to the faint; and to them that have no might he increaseth strength. Even the youths shall faint and be weary, and the young men shall utterly fall: But they that wait upon the LORD shall renew their strength; they shall mount up with wings as eagles; they shall run, and not be weary; and they shall walk, and not faint."

When you need God to pray for you

Romans 8:26-27 "Likewise the Spirit also helpeth our infirmities: for we know not what we should pray for as we ought: but the Spirit itself maketh intercession for us with groanings which cannot be uttered. And he that searcheth the hearts knoweth what is the mind of the Spirit, because he maketh intercession for the saints according to the will of God."

When you need grace

2 Corinthians 12:9-10 "And he said unto me, My grace is sufficient for thee: for my strength is made perfect in weakness. Most gladly therefore will I rather glory in my infirmities, that the power of Christ may rest upon me. Therefore I take pleasure in infirmities, in reproaches, in necessities, in persecutions, in distresses for Christ's sake: for when I am weak, then am I strong."

When everything seems impossible

Luke 1:37 "For with God nothing shall be impossible."

Philippians 4:13 "I can do all things through Christ which strengtheneth me."

When you're not sure how it will end

Jeremiah 29:11 "For I know the thoughts that I think toward you, saith the LORD, thoughts of peace, and not of evil, to give you an expected end."

When you need help from God

Psalm 18:1-3 "I will love thee, O LORD, my strength. The LORD is my rock, and my fortress, and my deliverer; my God, my strength, in whom I will trust; my buckler, and the horn of my salvation, and my high tower. I will call upon the

LORD, who is worthy to be praised: so shall I be saved from mine enemies."

When you are afraid

Psalm 27:1 "The LORD is my light and my salvation; whom shall I fear? the LORD is the strength of my life; of whom shall I be afraid?"

Psalm 56:3 "What time I am afraid, I will trust in thee."

Psalm 56:11 "In God have I put my trust: I will not be afraid what man can do unto me."

Isaiah 12:2 "Behold, God is my salvation; I will trust, and not be afraid: for the LORD JEHOVAH is my strength and my song; he also is become my salvation."